DR. ALAN HIRSCH SEPARATES SINUSITIS FACT FROM FICTION!

My cold has lasted more that one week. It must be a sinus infection.

In up to 25 percent of the cases, a cold lasts two weeks or more. . . . In other words, if you visit a doctor with a long-lasting cold (more than ten days) you may leave with a prescription for antibiotics for a diagnosed sinus infection. Unfortunately, that diagnosis and treatment could be wrong at least 25 percent of the time!

I snore every night and I have nasal congestion, so I probably have chronic sinusitis.

Snoring may indicate sinusitis, but the nasal congestion could be caused by asthma, allergies, or nasal obstruction associated with polyps or deviated septum.

I took a decongestant for my headache and it got better, so my pain must have been caused by a sinus headache.

This is generally not true. Nasal symptoms associated with colds and sinusitis generally do not resolve with decongestants and antihistamines that are designed to relieve symptoms only. However, these same medications usually relieve migraine pain.

BEFORE YOU POP THE PENICILLIN, PUT YOUR ASSUMPTIONS ASIDE AND CONSIDER . . .

WHAT YOUR DOCTOR MAY NOT TELL YOU ABOUT™ SINUSITIS

WHAT YOUR DOCTOR MAY *NOT* TELL YOU ABOUT™
SINUSITIS

Relieve Your Symptoms and Identify the *Real* Source of Your Pain

Alan R. Hirsch, M.D., F.A.C.P.

WARNER BOOKS

NEW YORK   BOSTON

The information herein is not intended to replace the services of trained health professionals. You are advised to consult with your health care professional with regard to matters relating to your health or the health of your child, and in particular regarding matters that may require diagnosis or medical attention.

WARNER BOOKS
Time Warner Book Group
1271 Avenue of the Americas, New York, NY 10020
Visit our Web site at www.twbookmark.com.

Printed in the United States of America

First Printing: May 2004

10 9 8 7 6 5 4 3 2 1

Library of Congress Cataloging-in-Publication Data

Hirsch, Alan R.
    What your doctor may not tell you about sinusitis : relieve your symptoms and identify the real source of your pain / Alan R. Hirsch.
        p. cm.
Includes bibliographical references and index.
    ISBN 0-446-69118-6
    1. Sinusitis.   I. Title.
    RF425.H55   2004
    616.2'12—dc22

2003022078

Book design by Charles A. Sutherland
Cover design by Diane Luger

For my beloved family:
Marissa, Jack, Camryn, Noah, and Debra

Acknowledgments

I could not have accomplished this book without the assistance of and help from many others.

Without the editorial style of my longtime friend, Virginia McCullough, and that of my editor at Time Warner, John Aherne, this book would have been, at best, incomprehensible. Thanks also to Noah Lukeman, of Lukeman Literary Agency, who conceived this project. Thanks to Dr. Jordan Pritikin of the Chicago Nasal and Sinus Center, and to my mentor, Dr. Joel Saper of the Michigan Head-Pain and Neurological Institute of Ann Arbor, Michigan, for their most valued input.

Thanks also to Dr. Jacob Fox, chairman of the Department of Neurology at Rush-Presbyterian-St.Luke's Medical Center in Chicago for his mentorship and steadfast support.

For her many years of devotion and effort, I wish to acknowledge Denise Fahey, practice administrator of the Smell and Taste Treatment and Research Foundation, Chicago.

Special thanks and love to my wife, Debra, and my children, Marissa, Jack, Camryn, and Noah, who generously sacrificed their time with me so that this book could be completed.

Alan R. Hirsch, M.D., F.A.C.P.
Neurological Director
Smell & Taste Treatment and Research Foundation
Chicago, Illinois

Contents

Foreword

The diagnosis and treatment of chronic sinusitis can at times be a daunting task. As a sinus specialist, I spend a large portion of my time seeing both patients who have been incorrectly diagnosed with chronic sinusitis, and patients with very subtle symptoms but with rather severe sinusitis. In fact, almost inexplicably, sinusitis appears to be at the same time both the most common chronic disease state and the most commonly *misdiagnosed* disease. These misdiagnoses occur at the hands of both patients and physicians alike.

Dr. Hirsch is highly respected in his field for work that sits at the crossroads of several specialties: neurology, psychiatry and otolaryngology (ears, nose, and throat). He has been an invaluable resource for a number of my patients, and I utilize his expertise for my patients who have refractory smell and headache problems. While it is true that Dr. Hirsch has published hundreds of articles in medical journals, it is his clinical acumen rather than his notable academic record that has continued to impress me.

In this text, Dr. Hirsch has done an outstanding job of explaining sinusitis and other disorders that may mimic sinusitis, including such common maladies as the common cold, allergies, migraine, and tension headaches. He does a wonderful job laying the foundation for these disease states, including their root causes, presenting symptoms and treatment options. This current text serves as an excellent resource for patients suffering from all of these disorders.

Jay M. Dutton, M.D.
Assistant Professor
Department of Otolaryngology
Rush University Medical Center
Chicago, IL

Introduction

—◦◦◦—

Sinusitis—A Diagnosis in Search of a Disease

In the late summer of 2002, a nineteen-year-old man living in Virginia went to see his family doctor complaining of fever, chills, fatigue, muscle aches, and sinus pain. He was diagnosed with acute sinusitis and given an antibiotic and another medication used to treat symptoms of sinus infections. The young man returned four days later with the same symptoms plus dizziness and nausea, along with a temperature of 103.5°F. On this visit the doctor performed some blood tests and after receiving the results, he changed the diagnosis to malaria. At that point, the treatment the young man received matched the diagnosis and he got well.

It is easy to see how a *mis*diagnosis, or a missed diagnosis, could occur. When the young man first went to his doctor no reason existed to believe he could have a disease like malaria. It's relatively rare in the United States and none of the risk factors—international travel, blood transfusions, and needle sharing—applied to him. No one among his immediate neighbors had developed the disease, although it was later discovered that he lived a half mile from another person who contracted malaria. This man lived within ten miles of the Washington-Dulles International Airport, which has nonstop flights from countries in which P-vivax malaria is endemic. After his diagnosis, mosquitoes were captured and tested within a few miles of his home and a small number (which is all that's needed to spread the disease) tested positive.

Am I saying that if you develop symptoms of sinusitis you should immediately consider malaria as a possibility and perhaps be tested for it prior to other treatment? No. Well, not exactly. You see, malaria represents only one, and fortunately rare, variation on the symptoms that can lead to a misdiagnosis of sinusitis. In 1992, malaria was considered eradicated from the United States, but since that time outbreaks have occurred and between 1,000 and 1,500 cases are reported every year, and it is likely many more have gone undiagnosed and unreported (or mistreated as sinusitis). So, yes, malaria is relatively rare, but because its symptoms mimic those of sinusitis, the initial misdiagnosis of the nineteen-year-old was considered important enough that JAMA (*Journal of the American Medical Association*) reported the case in November 2002. In other words, malaria, like many other common and much less esoteric diseases discussed in this book, cannot be taken off the list of possible conditions that produce the varied symptoms we associate with sinusitis.

I call sinusitis "a diagnosis in search of a disease" because much of the time, individuals develop a cluster of symptoms, some of which fit the criteria for a diagnosis of sinusitis. In the majority of cases, however, a diagnosis of sinusitis does not necessarily mean the person has sinusitis. Put another way, patients may leave their doctors' offices believing that the symptoms "add up" to sinusitis and they're relieved to have the label because most people tend to link a diagnosis with treatment whereby the condition will be cured. Unfortunately, the true cause of the symptoms could be allergic responses, common colds, headache syndromes, asthma, dental problems, nasal tumors, and even AIDS. The diagnostic line is blurry, especially when we attempt to differentiate a viral infection (the common cold) from a bacterial infection (that *may* be acute sinusitis), and distinguish sinusitis from migraine headaches.

A PICTURE OF CONFUSION

You can barely breathe, you can't smell the rolls in the bakery, and your face aches. You have sinusitis. Or do you? Given your symptoms, it is likely that sinusitis will be high on the list of possible diagnoses, should you see a doctor. Maybe this is not the first time you've had these symptoms and taken many trips to your doctor looking for an effective, lasting treatment. You may have seen several doctors in your quest for help.

Or maybe you have a history of frequent headaches. You also have nasal congestion, impaired ability to smell, and pain in your face, but you do not believe sinusitis is the cause of your symptoms. In fact, you never even thought about sinusitis and are not even sure what that means. To you, the symptoms are a sign that a migraine is on the way.

Or perhaps you have a cold that has lasted for two weeks and is draining your energy. You blow your nose all day, you cough, and your ears feel "stuffy." Although normally you don't go to the doctor with what you assume is a common cold, this time it's lasted so long that you make an appointment. What you may be told is that your viral infection (viral rhinitis) has become a bacterial sinus infection. You go home with an antibiotic and within a few days your symptoms may or may not begin to disappear. It seems logical to expect a cause-and-effect relationship between the antibiotic and the disappearance of the symptoms, but that expectation is not always scientifically sound.

Same symptoms, different cause, different treatments, and, perhaps most important, different "labels" may follow a patient around and start a cycle of incorrect treatments for a cluster of symptoms. Once a syndrome or a pattern of symptoms and diagnoses become part of a patient's medical history, this attached label often means that subsequent diagnoses will fall into similar patterns. Although many patients attempt to "start fresh," they find it a difficult task to accomplish.

Difficulty in achieving an accurate diagnosis is not an unusual situation in every branch of medicine. Unfortunately, some conditions lend themselves to confusion, and sinusitis is one of them. On the one hand, reported incidence of sinusitis is on the rise, but on the other hand, it is clear that this label could be incorrectly assigned to a group of symptoms not directly connected to the sinuses. The onset of a migraine headache can mimic some sinusitis symptoms, as can a long-lasting cold caused by a virus. Because so many symptoms overlap and treatments may be quite similar for a variety of conditions, medical professionals and patients end up confused.

Sadly, sinusitis symptoms don't involve just some isolated cases or a handful of situations in which an initial problem was misdiagnosed. Consider that between thirty-five and fifty million individuals (depending on what literature you read) are labeled as suffering from "sinus problems." Somewhere in the neighborhood of twenty million visits to doctors' offices take place annually because of sinus symptoms and most of these millions of patients leave with a prescription of some kind. It's a problem with huge dimensions and implications. Every day in my particular medical practice I see evidence that this is indeed an extremely confusing diagnostic situation.

THE DELICATE NOSE

The Smell & Taste Treatment and Research Foundation in Chicago sees more patients with smell and taste disorders (chemosensory impairment) than anywhere else in North America. About half the patients come from states outside Illinois, and approximately 25 percent come from other countries. On a daily basis patients are referred to the foundation with a diagnosis of sinusitis-induced smell loss. However, upon evaluation, this is almost never the case. The smell loss and headaches that are being attributed to sinusitis are instead due to other conditions that mimic sinusitis, a syndrome I call "pseudo-sinusitis." Studies have even suggested that if a patient comes to the doctor with a self-diagnosis of sinusitis, the diagnosis is incorrect about 98 percent of the time, and when a doctor diagnoses sinusitis, the diagnosis is incorrect about 90 percent of the time.

Clearly, the way to help relieve sinusitis-like symptoms is to treat the real problem. The word *sinusitis* literally means "inflammation of the sinuses." Though the term is used throughout this book, instead of sinusitis I probably should use the phrase "symptoms usually attributed to sinusitis but aren't really due to sinusitis." To clarify, I often use the terms *pseudo-sinusitis* and/or *sinusitis-like symptoms*.

Most of the time, the patients I see are motivated to seek help because of persistent sinusitis-like symptoms such as diminished, distorted, or (occasionally) increased ability to smell and taste. Almost always, I find other non-sinusitis conditions that result in these sinusitis symptoms, including headache syndromes—particularly migraines. Some of the same medications may work, at least temporarily, to relieve the symptoms of both sinusitis and non- or pseudo-sinusitis, but obviously an accurate diagnosis is in the patient's best interests.

It is unfortunate that loss of smell and taste are not considered major symptoms in the diagnosis of colds, allergies, nasal polyps, and sinusitis. I often see patients who have undergone years of treatment for sinus-related symptoms, and they may come to the Smell & Taste Treatment and Research Foundation because they have developed chemosensory impairment. Unfortunately, they frequently have lost the ability to smell and taste as a *result of the treatments* for the presumed sinusitis, and not necessarily because of the underlying disease.

Common prescription and over-the-counter medications such as nasal sprays and antihistamines may impair smell; in addition, surgery almost always affects this delicate sense. Surgery was once considered a valid and beneficial treatment, although smell loss often resulted, and quite often the loss was permanent. However, new thinking about the cause of sinus symptoms and sinusitis are radically changing attitudes toward surgery. In chapter 10 you will gain a better understanding of old and new thinking about sinus surgery.

This diagnosis-treatment confusion becomes more complex when we consider that the reported incidence of sinusitis is on the rise, but because it is likely *over*diagnosed, it may not be on the rise at all. If we misuse the term in the first place, more clusters of symptoms are likely to land under that diagnostic label.

Given the confusion about the matrix of symptoms that may be called "sinusitis," I've come to the conclusion that if you think you have sinusitis, you probably don't. About forty-five million cases of sinusitis are diagnosed each year; therefore, if even half of those diagnoses are incorrect it may result, at the very least, in massive amounts of unnecessary antibiotics. In actuality, the incidence of misdiagnosis is probably much higher. However, that doesn't mean you don't have nasal congestion, facial pain, and so forth. That just means you have some other condition that needs medical attention.

The reason it is important to read this book is to help you find treatment for the condition that is causing your sinusitis-like symptoms. The goal here is to understand sinusitis and to begin the process of determining if you truly have it or another condition, or a more complex combination of problems. In these pages, we will look at all the components of sinus disease, and we'll start by explaining the anatomy and physiology of the sinuses. The drawings should help you understand the origin of some symptoms, but may also help you to form relevant questions for your doctor. Equally important, this book can help you provide accurate answers to your doctor's questions. Accurate information can help guide diagnostic testing or correct previous misdiagnoses.

A WORD ABOUT "COST-EFFECTIVE TREATMENT"

The health care industry is greatly concerned about overall cost, and some treatment regimens are studied for cost in relation to treatment results for most of the patients most of the time. An article published in a medical journal in 2001 discussed treatment for acute sinusitis based on what is typically used in office-based medical practice. The article analyzed what treatments were cost effective on a *national* basis for the three million or so cases of acute bacterial sinusitis seen annually. For example, the study found that using X rays or CT scans to diagnose sinusitis has never been cost effective; on the other hand, antibiotics were. This means that based on presenting symptoms alone, diagnosing a sinus infection and giving the patient a prescription for an antibiotic is cost effective most of the time. However, the authors of the study point out that this inevitably leads to overuse of antibiotics, which as we now realize causes bacterial resistance and renders certain antibiotics ineffective over time. Antibiotics are becoming more expensive because of increased bacterial resistance—a growing global problem. Antibiotics also have side effects, which include vaginitis caused by overgrowth of yeast, gastrointestinal distress, and skin rashes.

Treating bacterial infections effectively with antibiotics means matching the drug with the bacteria causing the infection, which is why taking a culture is considered the "gold standard" method to diagnose a sinus infection. Culturing the sinuses is not considered cost effective, however, so the average patient is given one of the broad-spectrum antibiotics without a culture. Much of the time this works, insofar as the symptoms go away after the antibiotic is taken. However, just because symptoms disappear does not mean that an infection was present in the first place, nor does it mean the antibiotic helped the symptoms to go away.

An additional argument for treating virtually all patients who have what are widely believed to be symptoms of sinusitis is that acute sinusitis can have very rare but extremely serious complications. As the reasoning goes, if everyone with the symptoms of sinusitis is treated with antibiotics these complications will be largely avoided. At least half the prescriptions are given in error, however, which means millions of dollars of added cost, hardly cost-effective. And do we really want well over a million unnecessary antibiotic prescriptions written for just this one issue? Furthermore, there is no evidence that oral antibiotics actually prevent the progression of true sinusitis from the sinuses to the eyes or the brain. Again, the treatment is based on broad general diagnostic criteria, not on the diagnosis of individuals.

When you are ill you seek treatment as an individual and are not thinking about what is cost effective for society as a whole. In fact, as patients, we all have a responsibility to ask questions about the kind of medical advice we're given, precisely because we want to avoid such unnecessary medications as antibiotics. In addition, if the emphasis is on cost effectiveness, tests and procedures that might hasten the diagnostic process could be overlooked and a major problem could continue unnoticed.

I had a brush with erroneous cost-benefit analysis when as a new attending physician I suggested a complete battery of tests to narrow down the possible causes of the serious neurological symptoms of a particular patient. Rather than performing the tests, the intern tried different approaches that on the surface looked more compatible with the *probable* cause. Tragically, this resulted in months of unsuccessful treatment and incredible suffering, plus seven hospitalizations. Ultimately, one of the first tests I suggested was done and the diagnosis was finally made: arsenic poisoning. (It turned out a family member was poisoning the patient!) Not only was the piecemeal approach not cost effective in the long run, it extended the patient's suffering, which led to long-term problems. Of course, it also meant that the criminal in the family came close to getting away with murder. This goes to show why you have every right to insist on a complete diagnostic picture to avoid a one-size-fits-all sinusitis prescription.

The prescription for antibiotics given to treat your acute sinus infection may be based on statistics, presumed diagnosis, and treatment cost effectiveness, but not on your individual situation. We can always look at statistics for cost effectiveness, but we can't treat individual patients based on these numbers. It's like playing Russian roulette.

At this point I hope you can consider your condition with an open mind about the label that seems to fit but may not. Simply shifting your thinking away from the term *sinusitis* and to the term "sinusitis-like symptoms" opens the door to the possibility of a new way to view your condition.

Part I

DIAGNOSIS

Chapter 1

The Anatomy of Your Sinuses

Quite literally, sinuses are the holes—the cavities—inside the skull, specifically the air spaces around the nose and eyes. Sinuses exist in symmetrical sets or pairs. If you think of the center of your face as a square, the *frontal* sinuses are located in the upper two corners over the eyes in the forehead. The *maxillary* sinuses are located in the lower two corners next to your nose and extend down the upper cheeks and above the teeth. The *ethmoid* sinus cavities run along the side and back of your nose. (See figure 1.1.) This group of sinuses makes up the *paranasal* sinuses, so named because of their proximity to the nose. When we think of "stuffy" sinuses or sinus pain, these paranasal areas are most commonly involved, although as you will see, the pain itself does not necessarily originate in the sinuses. In addition, we have a pair of *sphenoid* sinuses located behind the eyes; these are the most deeply placed of the sinus cavities. Medical practitioners group the sinuses by pairs and think of eight separate structures. But these main sinus cavities contain other smaller ones, so we have approximately thirty

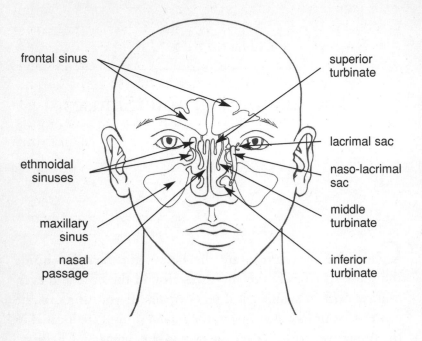

Figure 1.1 The septum.

sinus cavities that drain into the nose and form part of an efficient "drainage" system designed to help maintain health.

Each of these sinus pairs is connected to the nose through small openings called the *ostia* (the singular is ostium or "os"). The sinuses grow along with us; each sinus cavity is about the size of a pea in newborns, and will reach roughly walnut size by the time we're adults. A few people are born with one sinus cavity missing in a pair, and occasionally the frontal sinuses will not appear symmetrical. However, these abnormalities are not considered a cause of later sinus problems.

In addition to their role in helping to protect the body from potentially harmful invaders—viruses, fungi, and bacteria—sinuses also serve to lighten the skull. Some believe they act as mini shock absorbers, a mechanism designed to minimize damage from trauma to the face and head. The sinuses probably play a role in regulating pressure inside the nose and they may regulate the resonance of the voice. From an evolutionary point of view, the fact that the sinuses make the skull lighter may contribute to humans' ability to walk erect.

We cannot separate the nose and the sinuses because they are both covered by a membrane of mucus that resembles one long piece of plastic wrap. The nose is one end of the "wrap" and the sinuses form the other end. When we have a severe cold, the nose and sinuses are affected at the same time, so we should call a common cold *rhinosinusitis*, rather than simply *viral rhinitis*, as it is medically known.

FLOWING RIVERS AND DRAINAGE CANALS

The nose and sinuses work together to form one of the most important functions in the body, and while you may not think of your nose as a primary organ of the immune system, that's exactly what it is. When healthy, the sinuses are lined with mucus, a clear fluid that adds moisture to the air and warms it as you inhale. The mucosal lining is also part of the mechanism that processes odorant molecules and helps us detect scents in the air.

The sinuses contain *cilia*, tiny hair cells that propel or sweep mucus toward the openings (ostia) of the sinus cavities and into the nose. These cilia are always on the move as they cleanse the sinuses. Anything that slows or stops the sweeping motion of the cilia can cause stagnation and blockage in the sinuses, which then may develop into a sinus infection. (However, as discussed later, a "stuffy" nose is not necessarily a sign of an infection or a cold.) Unlike the clear, thin mucous discharge, yellow or green thickened discharge from the nose is a sign of sinus blockage, which makes the sinuses vulnerable to infections caused by viruses, bacteria, or fungi trapped in the sinus tissues. In addition, fluid buildup in the sinuses may cause pressure and pain. On the other hand, mildly blocked sinuses do not necessarily indicate the presence of a sinus infection.

In the maxillary sinuses, the ostium is located near the roof of the sinus and the cilia must work against gravity as they sweep upward to keep the river flowing. In a sense, the cilia have a tougher job—an "uphill battle"—and frequently are implicated in sinus infections. Inflammation tends to narrow the ostia and less oxygen reaches the sinuses and less foreign matter is cleared. This situation predisposes the sinuses to infection.

As an infection progresses, the mucosa (the lining) swells and the cavity may fill with pus. Over time, the chemistry of infected sinus cavities and the structure and chemistry of the cilia may change and when inflammation is chronic, irreversible scarring can occur. This situation also sets the stage for polyps to form. (Polyps are benign tissues that arise from the mucous membranes in the nose.) In addition, a sinus infection on one side can eventually spread to the opposing set of sinuses. In more than 40 percent of patients receiving a diagnosis of sinusitis, sinuses on both sides are affected. (This number would likely change if we were to weed out the cases of misdiagnosed sinusitis.)

The structures within the sinuses and nose are important because they form an "apparatus" that regulates the pathways for mucus to drain. Figure 1.1 shows the *septum*, which is made up of cartilage and bone, and is the structure that separates the two sides of the nose. We also have three bones, called *turbinates*, on the walls of the nose (see figures 1.2 and 1.3).

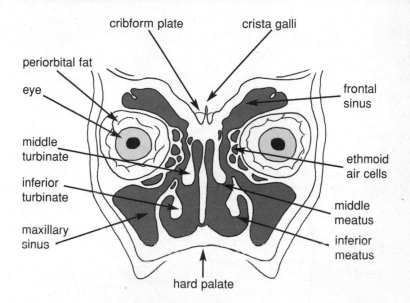

Figure 1.2 The sinuses.

The tear ducts in the corner of the eye (nasolacrimal ducts) drain beneath the lower turbinate. The frontal, ethmoid, and maxillary sinuses drain into the middle turbinate (see figure 1.4). The ethmoid sinuses in the back and sphenoid sinuses drain under the upper turbinate in the nose. Thus, all the sinuses ultimately drain into the nose.

Looking at figure 1.3, you can see the *nasopharynx*, the back of the nose, and the *eustachian tube*, which looks much like a piece of tubing between the nasopharynx and the ear. This connection is responsible for the sense of fullness in the ears when sinus blockages occur. We become conscious of the eustachian tube when air pressure changes on an airplane or in an elevator and we develop fullness or a stuffy feeling in our ears or experience a painful squeezing sensation. We can also feel ear fullness when problems in the sinuses cause nasopharyngeal inflammation.

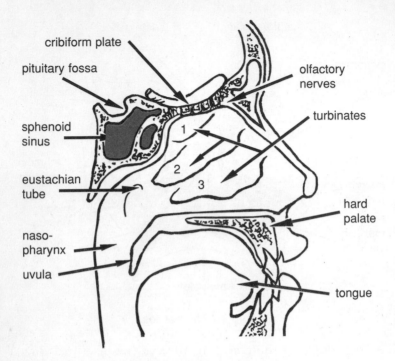

Figure 1.3 The nose.

The nasopharynx also contains lymph tissue, called the *adenoids*. Large adenoids can result in faulty sinus drainage. In infants, they are considered an important structure in the fight against infection, but the adenoids shrink as children become adults.

Dysfunction within any of the sinuses and the nasal structures can cause a variety of problems—from infection to blockages to breathing difficulties. However, many structural abnormalities are quite common and do not cause problems. For example, a condition such as *deviated septum* is defined as having a twist in the septum. Yes, this condition can cause blockages in the nat-

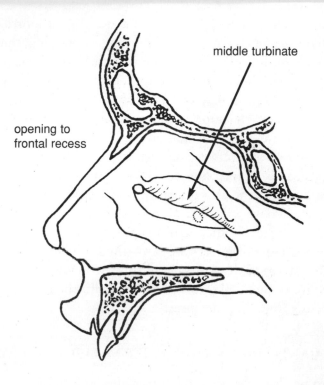

opening to
frontal recess

middle turbinate

Figure 1.4 The middle turbinate.

ural drainage system of sinuses and the nasal apparatus, but many people live with abnormalities of the septum and are not aware of it. Most physicians don't necessarily trace abnormalities that turn up on X rays or CT scans or magnetic resonance imaging (MRI) to diseases or conditions.

This situation is similar to what orthopedic specialists have discovered with the issue of back pain. A huge percentage of the population may have disk abnormalities, but many so-called abnormal individuals never suffer back pain, or they experience it only rarely. For many people back pain comes and goes and these individuals may or may not have abnormalities that show up on imaging tests. This may be puzzling, but over time orthopedic specialists concluded that structural abnormalities in the body do not automatically correlate to incidences of pain or disease or an eventual manifestation of any health problem. The same applies to structural deviations from what we consider the "normal nose."

In addition to sinuses and the "mechanical" parts of the nasal passages, twenty muscles in the upper airways regulate breathing, keep the airways open, and allow us to chew and swallow while we talk. Because so many diseases can produce symptoms involving the nasal structures and sinuses, it is easy to see why exact diagnoses are sometimes difficult to make. In addition, these intricate nasal and sinus structures are part of a protective system designed to keep us well. The nose is one of the body's "first-line" defenses.

CILIA AND MUCUS: OUR BUILT-IN LIFE PRESERVERS

Just to be clear, the nose, nasal passages, and sinuses are lined with a wet "wrap" we call the *mucous membrane*, which in turn produces mucus. The nose and sinuses act to regulate the flow of mucus in the body, and we produce and drain an average of a quart of mucus every day. We swallow it, we remove it when we blow our nose, and it also evaporates. The normal sinus and nasal drainage systems are like a river of mucus that flows freely, and when working well, this river is an important component of what protects us from illness. The whole system works to preserve and protect life, and we can think of the nose as a hero that employs mucus as one of its major weapons.

The sticky mucus produced in the nose traps infectious agents. The nasal airway bends at about a ninety-degree angle at the nasopharynx, where it traps even more "invaders." These invaders sometimes become stuck on the wall—much like flies on flypaper.

We may release these invading agents when we sneeze or they may drain in the mucus down the back of the throat. We swallow the mucus continually, and the bacteria, viruses, and fungi are destroyed in the gastrointestinal (GI) system. The GI tract is one of the body's primary infection fighters. Keep in mind that this river of mucus flows fast, moving mucus at the rate of six or seven millimeters a minute. (My kids have fun thinking of this mucus like the "canal of slime" in the movie *Ghostbusters 2*. They tease me and say I'm like an explorer in the "river of snot." Even Oprah once referred to me as "the Magellan of the nasal passages!")

Nasal secretions also contain particular enzymes (*lysozymes*) that help break down and destroy the invading particles. These secretions also contain antibodies that act directly against invading bacteria. Just as we have beneficial bacteria in the GI tract, however, we have beneficial bacteria in the nasal structures, too. Although I clarify this issue in chapter 5 when I discuss new theories about sinus problems, it is important to keep in mind that all bacteria aren't the "enemy."

The river of mucus can slow down for many reasons, some of which are benign and normal responses to internal or external stimuli or invaders. Stuffy noses, watery eyes, thick yellow or green mucus, and so forth can be temporary conditions or they can be symptoms of colds, sinusitis, allergies, asthma, and headache. Blockages in the sinuses do not cause sinusitis, but they may slow down the normal drainage process and set the stage for sinus problems to develop. When it comes to respiratory health, the most important goal we can have is to keep the mucus river flowing in order to avoid stagnation and sluggish movement.

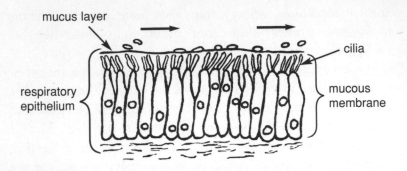

Figure 1.5 Cilia.

The mucosal surface in the nose is a vascular area, meaning that it contains an intricate system of blood vessels. Irritants and foreign particles can cause engorgement and the flushing effects of mucus, or in more common terms, a runny nose. For example, cigarette smoke is an irritant and can slow down the cleansing effects of cilia as they try to push mucus through the nasal structures. When working normally, the cilia have phases: in one phase, they beat rapidly and stand up straight; in another phase they bend in the opposite direction and move more slowly. Rapid movement of the cilia keep infectious agents out of the sinuses. Anything that slows them down increases the chances for infection (by viruses or bacteria) or for obstruction.

Cilia are the unsung heroes of the breathing apparatus and of the protective mechanism of the nose and the river of mucus (see figure 1.5). In addition to cigarette smoke, several other "everyday" conditions and substances can damage or hamper the work of the cilia. These include cold temperatures, dry air, and iced drinks, along with common drugs such as antihistamines and codeine. Although it is not an "everyday" issue, the well-documented damage that cocaine does to the nose involves damage to the cilia. In addition, toxins such as formaldehdye, chromium dust, and chlorine gas also potentially damage cilia. Anything that damages cilia through trauma, irritation, or by drying action may potentially compromise their protective function, leaving the body more susceptible to infection. Protecting your cilia is a good reason to avoid situations that compromise their function. Those with sinusitis-like symptoms must be especially careful to avoid anything that further slows the movement of the cilia.

THE TURBINATES: A CLOSER LOOK

The turbinates (see figure 1.3) also have a daily life-preserving function because they filter the air as you inhale and trap invaders. Any number of conditions cause swelling in the turbinates, which you may experience as nasal obstruction that worsens when you're lying down. This happens because fluid and blood tend to pool in the head when you're reclining.

Even while you sleep the turbinates help regulate the movement of fluid in your body. You turn or move around about fifty times during a normal sleep cycle. When you're sleeping on your right side, gravity causes the right turbinates to fill. Eventually, they fill to the point of pressure on the septum, which you respond to by turning over on the other side and the cycle starts again. Moving around while you sleep moves lymph fluid through the body and keeps the blood moving in your veins, thus protecting you from "hemostasis," which literally means "blood staying still." To illustrate, consider that the turbinates are one of the body's mechanisms that protect you from stroke, because pressure on them triggers you to move around. This movement prevents blood from pooling in your veins (*venostasis*), thus preventing blood clots (which could cause a stroke) from forming. Thus, the sensation of the turbinates filling with fluid literally helps you survive because it causes you to move and protects you from the risks associated with lack of movement.

Since your level of sleep changes throughout the night, you rouse just enough to move, although you generally do not become conscious of the pressure that caused you to turn. You usually sleep through these natural phases. On the other hand, a deviated septum may prevent the normal sensation of pressure during sleep, thereby causing a deeper level of sleep, which reduces the amount of oxygen that reaches the tissues. A form of sleep apnea occurs when the oxygen level drops to the point that the sleeper snorts, often loudly enough to "shock" the body into moving and relieving the pressure on the turbinate. (Many causes of sleep apnea exist; this is just one of the possible mechanisms.) So, along with cilia and mucus, the structures of the nose represent another life-preserving mechanism. We could say that the turbinates are on "watch" every night.

THE REAL SITE OF SINUS PAIN

You have probably seen commercials for over-the-counter (OTC) remedies for "sinus headaches." One reason for confusion about headaches and sinusitis is that on the commercials, a person is seen pinching the nose or forehead, and touching the area around the nose or eyes. Logically, people think that since the eyes and nose are close, and sinuses are around the eyes, it must be a sinus headache. Despite what we have been led to believe, the sinuses are not the source of the pain. Rather, the source is located inside the nose, not the sinuses.

It's important to understand that pain is not always felt at the source of stimulation. Conventional medical thinking holds that if you stimulate the nasal turbinates, you produce pain around the eyes (infraorbital region) and the cheek. Stimulating the inside of the nose at the location where the sinuses drain (the ostia) produces pain around the eyes and forehead and the middle of the head. It is said that stimulating the ethmoid sinuses produces pain on the top of the head, and if you stimulate the sphenoid sinuses the pain is experienced on the front, side, and back of the head, and around and above the eye. The pain can occur on one (unilateral) or both (bilateral) sides. If the person has any engorged nasal mucosa or inflammation while being stimulated, the pain can become more intense and spread farther. Thus, where you feel pain is *not* necessarily where the disease is located.

In an experiment that "mapped" pain patterns, a balloon was inserted into the maxillary sinuses through a cavity left by tooth extraction. Then the balloon was inflated, producing only moderate pain. The pain from the "balloon" experiment developed slowly, but the pain produced by electrically stimulating the sinus ostia (the openings of the sinuses located in the nose) produced rapidly developing pain. The implication is that the sinuses themselves are relatively insensitive to swelling and pain, as compared to the structures of the nose. If you put pressure on the maxillary sinuses, it's not painful, but pain is produced if pressure is placed on the ostia of the sinuses and the nasal turbinates. Thus, what people think of the pain of sinusitis doesn't involve the structures of the sinuses themselves. Sinus pain really means "sinus ostium pain" or "nasal turbinate pain." Even pain experienced from true sinusitis originates from the ostia, which are only the sinus openings, not the sinuses themselves.

If we electrically stimulate the nasal mucosa, pain can be felt in the neck and the shoulders. This situation is related to the phenomenon of *referred pain*, which is caused by intermingling of nerve fibers. This stimulation pattern helps explain why people with neck and shoulder pain could have dysfunction of the nasal turbinates. This is similar to misdiagnosing a migraine as sinusitis because the areas of pain are misunderstood. In essence, we may overlook dysfunction of the turbinates and ostia and treat neck and shoulder pain as an isolated event.

With pain in the sinuses, as in what we casually label a sinus headache, we usually see an inflammatory reaction along with swelling of the nasal mucosa. It seems that this inflammation produces blockage (*occlusion*) of one (or more) of the sinus ostia. The inflammation may also increase pressure on the mucosa of the nasal turbinate. This swelling is more likely to occur if there is a deviation of the nasal septum or an abnormality that narrows the nasal cavity. (Nasal swelling also is involved with the olfactory cycle, explained in chapter 7.)

Think of the area next to the middle turbinate (see figure 1.4) as a canal that receives drainage from the tear ducts and three sinus pairs: maxillary, frontal, and ethmoid. If the mucosa swells, blockage can occur in any of the drainage areas or "ducts," which then allows fluid to accumulate and form what we can descriptively call a "swamp" or "pond" conducive to bacterial growth. An allergic reaction can produce swelling in this area, too.

To sum up the results of pain location research, it appears that the sinus ostia and turbinates are susceptible to pain, not the sinus cavities themselves. In addition, pain is not caused by fluid in the sinuses. Understanding this explains why X rays and CT scans show the fluid, but the patient may not experience pain. Conversely, the presence of the fluid in the sinuses doesn't explain why the individual is having pain; irritation of the ostia and nasal turbinates, not the sinuses, causes the pain. What we currently call "sinus pain" should probably be renamed "turbinitis," meaning inflammation of the nasal turbinates. Keep in mind that sinusitis pain is not caused by fluid in the cavities, and pain associated with sinus conditions may be referred pain experienced in the neck and shoulders. Other causes of pain in these sinus regions exist, but for now, it's important to understand that fluid in the sinuses is not a direct cause of what has become known as a sinus headache. Nor does pain around the sinuses mean that an infection is present.

When you continue with the rest of the information presented in this book, keep in mind the following points:

1. Sinus symptoms can be caused by a wide variety of conditions.
2. The river of mucus acts as a protective mechanism, always working to protect the body from infection.
3. Pain experienced in the sinuses is usually not due to disease in the sinuses themselves.
4. Sinusitis is a misnomer, and as a distinct infection, it is probably over- and misdiagnosed. Pseudo-sinusitis syndrome or sinusitis-like symptoms may better describe the cluster of symptoms that are routinely labeled sinusitis.

Chapter 2

Cold Symptoms or
Sinusitis Symptoms?

Although many conditions can cause stagnation in what I have called "the river of mucus," for the sake of clarity, let's look at the way sinusitis is *currently* clinically defined and classified. Then we can contrast it with other conditions that produce the same symptoms to gain a better understanding about why sinusitis can be so easily misdiagnosed. I put emphasis on the word *currently* because new information will likely change the definitions and classifications over time.

Sinusitis is classified as acute, subacute, or chronic, depending on its duration. *Acute* sinusitis generally lasts no more than four weeks; *sub-acute* sinusitis lasts from four to twelve weeks, and if the infection lasts more than twelve weeks, it is considered *chronic*. Sinusitis may be considered chronic if the infections occur more than four times a year. No hard and fast rule exists about how many infections per year define chronic, because some infections may linger on and some individuals have several separate infections over a period of months. However, these time frames are based on generally accepted classifications issued by the AAO–HNS (American Academy of Otolaryngology–Head and Neck Surgery). They are arbitrary in the sense that they help define the characteristics of the condition, but are based *only* on time, and not any aspect or feature of the disease itself, such as symptoms, origin, or progression. This is why many physicians have rejected these classifications. In medicine, this type of classification is necessary in order to discuss a condition and a set of symptoms, but it may not be helpful in assessing individual cases.

Symptoms that *may* be associated with sinusitis include:

- stuffed-up nose (congestion), or green or yellow nasal mucus, which indicates that the discharge is coming from the sinuses into the nose
- facial pain, which may include pressure or pain that starts on one side of the face, or that worsens when leaning forward, or a feeling of fullness in the face or around the eyes, even in the absence of pain
- fever (at the onset of acute sinusitis)
- impaired smell and flavor
- headache
- an ache in the upper teeth
- halitosis
- fatigue/malaise
- cough
- pain, pressure, or a feeling of fullness in the ears

A patient once said that sinusitis is a "draining disease," which is literally true, of course. However, he meant that it sapped his strength and made every day an effort. Any of the symptoms listed can make life unpleasant, at the very least. For many reasons, it is not an easy condition to learn to live with, not the least of which is that it often interrupts sleep. Chronic sinusitis is especially emotionally draining because those affected may not see an end in sight. This is made worse when the diagnosis is questionable.

Many things can trigger a sinus infection. These include:

- colds and upper respiratory infections. Sinusitis may occur when a common cold appears to be getting better, then takes a turn for the worse.
- allergies and hay fever. (Sometimes these conditions can be confused with sinusitis.)
- immune conditions, such as diabetes or AIDS, which can cause chronic sinusitis because of persistent fungal infections
- aging, which is an independent factor. The chances of developing sinusitis increase with age.
- hormonal changes, particularly at puberty and pregnancy
- air travel or swimming underwater, both of which can cause a change in the air pressure that blocks the sinuses
- any kind of nasal procedure or surgery and dental work
- air pollution, including cigarette smoke
- coughing and sneezing and even the pressure from having a bowel movement can cause sinusitis
- trauma and injury

As you can see, the symptoms and the causes are quite extensive. Ironically, this is both good news and bad news. Certainly, the symptoms are common and virtually every family physician sees them on a regular basis. In fact, conditions that can be characterized by "nasal congestion" and all its offshoots are probably among the "original" medical conditions suffered by early human beings on the planet. However, because the symptoms are so common and varied, the term *sinusitis* itself has come into popular usage and has lost some of its specific meaning, even among many doctors. In other words, a person may have a cold, but because the sinuses drain, he or she calls the cold sinusitis. The misuse of the term has occurred for many reasons, but in order to straighten out the confusion, we need to begin with symptoms.

HOW A SINUS INFECTION DIFFERS FROM A COLD

Since sinus infections are often linked with the common cold, let's look at what a cold is and what it isn't. First, colds appear to be an accepted annoyance of the human condition. Ancient Chinese and Greek medical texts refer to them, but often in a positive way, because they were viewed as the body's natural process of cleansing. In modern language, we might call this "detoxification." Indeed, even today if you see a Chinese medical practitioner or a naturopathic doctor (one of the alternative health care practitioners) you might be reassured that your symptoms are a sign that the body is clearing toxins from your system. If that's true, there's a considerable amount of "detoxing" going on because more than 150 million people contract colds (or demonstrate cold symptoms) annually. Having about two colds a year is considered average. In terms of lost work and school time, each year, colds are responsible for about 440 million days absent from the office or factory and 62 million days away from school.

In conventional Western medicine, colds are viewed as an illness in which patients feel lousy and want to get rid of the symptoms as soon as possible. In addition, because viruses cause them, colds aren't viewed as the body's attempt to do anything positive. The medical term for a cold is *rhinovirus*, which literally means virus of the nose. (When you hear "rhino" you know it involves the nose.) The rhinovirus is only one of 125 known viruses that may cause a cold. Because so many different viruses are responsible for common colds and related symptoms, developing a vaccine has to date been impossible. In addition, a person can have a cold caused by one virus and still be susceptible to a cold caused by another.

WORKING DEFINITION OF RHINOVIRUS OR COLD

Colds have been classified in terms of duration, although again, these classifications may or may not be of any relevance for individuals. In fact, the overclassification of symptoms related to colds may lead to overtreatment or unnecessary treatment. This occurs in part because the symptoms of a cold and sinusitis are so similar.

Our first reaction to cold symptoms is usually to groan and say we don't have time for this. We usually feel put upon—the "why me" response. But unless we live in a sanitized bubble, we live in a virtual swamp of viruses and bacteria, which are passed around in various ways. Schools and workplaces are filled with people who sneeze and cough and otherwise pass around cold viruses. Any place where people congregate is a place to "catch a cold," which is how we generally think of the transmission. Frequent hand washing is one of the best ways to prevent the spread of cold viruses when you are exposed to an extra dose of the "swamp." Teachers, day care workers, and so forth are frequently exposed and must take care to avoid infection.

Common cold—rhinovirus—symptoms include:

- dryness or irritation in the throat. (This may be your first symptom.)
- clogged or stuffy nose (to varying degrees), watery discharge
- a feeling of heaviness in the sinuses—areas in the face, forehead, around the eyes
- fullness in the ears
- headache
- sore throat
- mild cough
- smell and taste impairment

Less common symptoms include:

- low-grade fever
- varying degrees of fatigue and malaise
- muscle aches

In contrast, true acute sinusitis is actually quite rare and is usually seen in people who are immunocompromised, such those with unstable diabetes or those with AIDS. Acute sinusitis develops in susceptible individuals.

WHY IS WINTER "COLD SEASON"?

We tend to think of winter as "cold season," which isn't true. September is a peak month for colds among children, and summer colds are as common as winter colds among adults. However, immunity does fluctuate seasonally. Most parents nag their children to dress warmly, to keep their hats on and jackets zipped, and to take off wet clothes immediately. They say this with the warning that "you'll catch cold" if you are exposed to "the elements." For years now, conventional wisdom has rendered our parents' warnings as nothing more than old wives' tales. Viruses cause colds, not wet feet or wet hair or cold air. Although it's true that viruses cause colds, the old wives' tales do have scientific basis.

White blood cells (*lymphocytes*) help destroy incoming viruses and bacteria, an essential function of the immune system. Immunity tends to be more repressed in lower temperatures than higher temperatures, so winter is a risk in that sense. Staying warm helps maintain immunity to potentially harmful viruses and bacteria, so anything that gives your immune system a boost to better do its job is helpful. So, while I don't recommend making an emergency out of becoming wet and chilled, I don't think parents are silly for nagging their kids about staying warm. Besides, it's advice all adults should take seriously.

Whether or not a person develops a cold comes down to immune system function, or put another way, the condition of the "host." A virus invades a host and if immunity is strong, the virus doesn't stand a chance. Some people seldom contract colds because for some reason their particular immune system is "hardy." When these individuals do develop a cold it may be mild and of short duration.

Immunity is a complex issue and will come up from time to time in this book. But here, let me say that the immune system is not one system, but many systems, and multiple factors are involved in keeping the body free of infectious disease. Furthermore, we are only beginning to understand the cause of illness in any individual at any given time. Still, the conventional wisdom that we are susceptible to colds when we're "run down," a nonspecific term if there ever was one, does indeed contain some truth. You probably know firsthand that when you are stressed, tired, overworked, or emotionally upset, or when your lifestyle is "out of whack" for some reason, you are more likely to develop a cold. (And because you're under excessive stress, you say it's the worst possible time.) Numerous studies demonstrate the effects of stress on the immune system and without question, that run-down feeling is real; avoiding colds is one of several reasons to make sure you eat well, get adequate rest, and so on. This is truly common sense.

As stated previously, in the United States, September is a peak month for colds, so winter isn't cold season after all. This peak is believed to be due to children returning to school, thus increasing their exposure to many more children who are incubating any number of cold viruses.

WHY A COLD MAY BE SIGNIFICANT TO SINUSITIS

Colds become dangerous if they develop into other infections, such as bronchitis, pneumonia, or sinus infections, or when these infections are bacterial in origin. Some sinus infections are bacterial in nature, which is why they may respond to antibiotics. The reason the sinus infection may develop is related to the function of the "the river of mucus." Cold viruses cause the nasal passages to swell because the body fights the invader by increasing blood circulation to the area. As a defense mechanism, the runny discharge helps to fight the viral invasion. When mucus flow is stalled or slows down (because of swelling in the nasal cavity, for example), the stage is set for possible infection because stagnation in the sinuses stops the normal flow of mucus and turns into a breeding ground for bacteria. This is how a viral cold sometimes turns into a bacterial sinus infection. To try to keep the river of mucus flowing, stay away from smoke and drink plenty of water to stay well hydrated. In addition, do not use antihistamines because they dry the sinus cavities, which further slows the river of mucus.

In general, colds run their course, and whether treated or not they last a week to ten days; however, in up to 25 percent of the cases, a cold lasts two weeks or more. This may seem confusing, but a criterion for a sinus infection is a cold that has lasted longer than ten days. In other words, if you visit a doctor with a long-lasting cold (more than ten days) you may leave with a prescription for antibiotics for a diagnosed sinus infection. Unfortunately, that diagnosis and treatment could be wrong at least 25 percent of the time! In fact, it is probably wrong much more often than that because of the faulty definition of sinusitis in the first place.

FIGHTING YOUR SYMPTOMS

Treating a cold with OTC symptom-relief medications is about trying to feel better rather than speeding up recovery. However, giving your body the optimal conditions to get over a cold may help prevent a later sinus infection (or a lingering cold) because there is a slight chance that an extended cold may develop into sinusitis. Drink fluids such as tea and hot soup and consume adequate water. These fluids help keep the mucus flowing through the nose, which clears the infected material. A runny nose is annoying, but it is a cleansing mechanism and helps prevent the stagnation that creates a favorable environment for a sinus infection.

Twenty-five years ago, a study suggested that chicken soup really does help a cold because it increases mucus flow in the nose. I'm not sure if anyone has replicated the findings, but, for some reason, chicken soup has a folklore quality now, and since most of us probably believe it's the best broth for fighting colds, maybe it is because of the placebo effect. The important element is that clear liquids keep mucus flowing, which is why increasing fluid intake is one of the best self-care measures you can take. In addition to increasing fluids, you should cut back on activity, and if your symptoms are severe, stay home and rest. (I realize this is difficult for many people because "working sick" is the norm in many offices and factories.) When you have a severe cold, your body aches and the combination of symptoms may make you so tired that you can't work, so attempting to do so is foolish.

In addition, a well-humidified environment is best because the cilia (the tiny hairs in your respiratory system) do a better job of cleansing the nose in a moist atmosphere. Moist air also keeps the mouth from becoming dry. A room humidifier or a central system allows water particles into the air, and the moisture is the same temperature as the air in the room.

Vaporizers produce steam by converting the water into a gas—water vapor—thereby filling the area with steam. Some people find this soothing. The aromatic products you can use in a vaporizer do not necessarily have a medicinal benefit, but they may be pleasant and make you feel better because you like the scent. (More on that later.) Vaporizers involve hot water that could burn if spilled, so be cautious about their use in your child's room. If you use a humidifier, be sure to regularly wash out the water reservoir so that fungi do not build up in that optimal breeding environment.

Should you blow your nose frequently, or should you sniff back to clear your nose? Gently blowing your nose, with one or both nostrils open, is safe and relieves discomfort. Conversely, blowing hard while pressing on both sides of your nose is potentially dangerous. Blowing hard can push secretions to the back of the nose and into the eustachian tubes, in which case, an ear infection can develop. So the goal in blowing your nose is to clear secretions out, not force them back. Use tissues rather than a cloth handkerchief, which is a breeding ground for the very viruses from which you're trying to recover. Sniffing also is a safe way to clear the nose and is not a cause of a sinus infection.

A cough is usually a normal part of a cold, and often has beneficial effects, because it helps clear cold secretions from your bronchial tubes and windpipe. In this case, you don't want to keep the cough suppressed all day because it has a helpful job in recovering from a cold and preventing other infections. Coughs are annoying, however, and staying well hydrated will help. OTC cough drops or cough medication may ease the irritation, especially if a cough is interfering with sleep. Some people find that a spoonful of honey soothes a sore throat and mild cough.

A cough that becomes hacking or that produces thick mucus that is hard to loosen or raise can become "violent" and even fracture the ribs or rupture a blood vessel in the head. In this situation, suppressing the cough may be protective, but violent coughing may indicate a worsening infection, including pneumonia. While a cough can "hang on" for a few days after a cold has run its course, a persistent, nagging cough is associated with many illnesses and conditions and should always be investigated by a physician. A chronic cough may be a side effect of some medications, so do not ignore it.

HOLD THE ANTIBIOTICS

Remember: Colds are not sinus infections, even though the sinuses are involved symptomatically. Bacteria cause many sinus infections, which is why antibiotics may be effective in some cases; however, antibiotics are not effective for cold viruses. When they are used for the wrong application, antibiotics can interfere with healing. As previously stated, overuse of antibiotics has led to a rapidly growing problem of bacterial resistance.

In addition, colds are not hay fever or allergies, although the symptoms may overlap. Common colds, hay fever, and allergies can lead to a sinus infection, but the congestion associated with an allergy is not synonymous with sinusitis, and impaired smell and taste associated with colds is not necessarily the result of sinusitis.

SELF-CARE AND HOME TREATMENTS

Instead of, or in addition to, using OTC medications, some people turn to vitamins or herbal preparations, most of which do not have significant side effects and will not cause drowsiness or otherwise interfere with daily life. For example, ever since Linus Pauling, the Nobel Prize–winning scientist, wrote extensively about vitamin C and colds, some people swear that taking the vitamin will shorten the duration of a cold. But studies have not produced definitive results, and taking vitamin C appears to be more a matter of belief and personal preference. In addition, many "hard-core" believers say that the vitamin does not have a significant effect on the course of a cold, but its action to enhance immune system function does give it a role in preventing colds, rather than in treating them.

Beyond vitamins, some substances have been shown to play a role in immunity, specifically in relation to colds. For example, in recent years, garlic has been touted as an immune system stimulant, and as having antibacterial and antiviral properties. The herb *Echinacea purpurea* has a long history as an herbal remedy and it is said to increase the body's white blood cells, thereby fighting infection, so it, too, is purported to stimulate immunity. The herb goldenseal is said to strengthen weakened membranes in the nose. A homeopathic cold remedy, *Oscillococcinum*, is available in this country and is widely used in Europe. (To date, studies of homeopathic cold remedies have not demonstrated any degree of efficacy.)

Without question, dozens, if not hundreds, of herbal cold preparations exist in this country and across the globe, but I am unable to recommend any of them. In addition, I cannot recommend any of the remedies that fall under the umbrella of "natural," even though they may have merit and are used throughout the world. There are several reasons for this.

First, most of the natural remedies have not come under scientific investigation (at least by standards used in the United States and approved by the Federal Drug Administration), so I can't state that they have a valid place in treatment. In addition, herbs come in capsule form, as teas, or as tinctures (diluted in alcohol or water). Because their production is not regulated, these herbal preparations aren't prepared and packaged under uniform standards. In addition, optimal dosages as well as the source of the herbs are unknown. I have read reports of high levels of lead neurotoxic metal in some herbal preparations.

Even vitamin C comes in many different forms and its quality varies. Most doctors (in every specialty) trained in the United States are not educated about these remedies and therefore do not use them in their practices. In recent years, however, we have become aware of them because patients ask about them or tell us that they use them. In many cases, they are part of what we now call "integrative medicine."

Does this mean that I am telling you not to use herbal or nutritional remedies? Of course not, and in fact, I discuss some nonconventional therapies in this book. But I do advise you to seek advice from doctors who are knowledgeable and trained in the safe use of these products (e.g., vitamin C and plant remedies, including garlic). So, if you are interested in Chinese herbal medicine (or practices such as acupuncture), seek the services of a doctor trained in Chinese medicine and who is established in your community. Nowadays, many communities across the United States have doctors experienced in some aspect of integrative medicine, from herbal remedies and nutritional therapies to acupuncture and biofeedback. Consult these professionals and never rely on untrained practitioners and health food store employees for advice about the safe use of nutrients and herbs.

"Natural" remedies for colds, sinus congestion, and other illnesses are often said to be "safe," but natural is not synonymous with safe, precisely because these products are not standardized and their quality is not controlled. (See the nasal spray example that follows.) Hence, even though we live in a time with vast choices in health care, patients still have a great responsibility to investigate any therapy they are offered, including natural remedies.

THE RISK OF OVERMEDICATING

There are numerous OTC cold medications that represent a huge industry. These medications are considered safe, although they, too, may have problems associated with them. One reason sinusitis and colds are confused with each other is that advertising for OTC cold and allergy medications may claim that they relieve many symptoms associated with both colds and sinusitis (such as Advil Cold and Sinus), and these symptoms overlap with allergies. Adding the term *sinusitis* to a label leads to increased self-diagnosis and also implies that the presence of cold symptoms plus headache and/or facial pain somehow adds up to sinusitis. This leads to inaccurate or "loose" definitions of the condition.

Most cold medications found in drugstores and supermarkets usually are a combination of drugs that may include an antihistamine, a decongestant, a cough suppressant, and an analgesic. Of course, you may not need any of these drugs, and these symptomatic remedies do not make your cold go away any faster. Many people don't take them at all, and find that rest and liquids do about as well. (See the list of medications and side effects in the appendix.)

Antihistamines. These are not particularly useful for the common cold, which is caused by a virus. Antihistamines are typically used for allergy symptoms and as such, they have a drying effect on the nasal passages. But this drying effect also tends to thicken the mucus in the nose and throat, which increases the risk that the sinuses will become "plugged" and/or the eustachian tube blocked. Thus, it's best to avoid cold medications with antihistamines because they may increase your risk of developing a sinus infection.

In addition, these OTC antihistamines can cause drowsiness. If you do use them for any reason, do not drive or operate machinery. For certain, if your job involves using mechanical or electrical equipment, do not take these antihistamines.

Decongestants. The oral decongestant preparations treat congestion by opening the nose and shrinking the nasal passages. Some are available without any of the other "ingredients" and are safe for the common cold. Although they are nonprescription drugs, *I recommend asking your doctor if they are safe in your case because individuals with cardiovascular problems, hypertension, thyroid conditions, glaucoma, and men with prostate disease shouldn't use them.* This covers millions of individuals, which is why they shouldn't be considered safe across the board. Some decongestants include a cough suppressant, so if they are safe in your case, your cough may be manageable as well.

Analgesics. This is the umbrella term for painkillers such as aspirin or acetaminophen—standard OTC pain relievers. They have no effect on nasal symptoms, but may relieve headaches or muscle aches.

Zinc lozenges. In recent years, zinc gluconate lozenges have been shown to reduce the severity and length of a cold. Some people say that if they take the zinc lozenges at the first sign of a cold, it often won't develop at all or will be mild. Zinc has been said to have a positive effect on the immune system, so it makes sense that it could provide the body what it needs to fight off the invading virus. However, the most recent information questions this theory and proposes that zinc actually acts to harm the body by suppressing immune system function, thus promoting infection. Ask your doctor about zinc before using it in lozenge form. (Taking zinc in tablet form does not have the same effect as the lozenge.) Some of the flavorings that mask the unpleasant taste of the zinc may render it inactive, so ask your doctor for a recommendation on the type of zinc to use and ask for advice about the dosage. Zinc is a powerful mineral, but it works synergistically with other minerals in the body, so taking too much can disrupt the necessary balance. The correct amount is safe but too much may cause trouble. To use these lozenges properly they must be dissolved in the mouth and not chewed or swallowed. Some people experience mouth irritation or the taste is too unpleasant to tolerate.

BE CAREFUL WITH NASAL SPRAYS—
ESPECIALLY ZINC

Nasal sprays have been used extensively, particularly by the many millions of individuals who have risk factors that limit decongestant use. They open the nasal passages by relieving the swelling that occurs in the lining of the nose during a cold. Many are available without prescription, but their use should be restricted to no more than four days. Unfortunately, many people casually buy these sprays in the drugstore and are unaware that they can become addicted. This occurs because the user seeks the relief the spray delivers and, when the symptoms return, uses the spray again. The tissues shrink and swell, each time producing a "rebound" effect, which means that the medication loses effectiveness, must be used more frequently, and ultimately, the user becomes dependent on it and reaches for it as soon as the congestion returns. The only "cure" is to quit using the product altogether, which means going through a withdrawal period in which the nasal passages remain swollen. For this reason, stop using *any* spray after the *fourth* day. In addition, I recommend avoiding steroid nasal sprays (available by prescription), because the steroid medication may depress the immune system and further entrench the cold.

Earlier I mentioned that natural products might or might not be safe. One example is a nasal spray called Zicam. In a relatively short period of time, I saw a cluster of patients who had used the spray and then lost their sense of smell. Zinc has long been known to cause smell loss. During the polio epidemic it was believed that the polio virus was spread through inhalation and some physicians believed that zinc would damage olfactory ability and thus prevent the virus from entering the nose. They further believed this would prevent the spread of polio in the population. Parents put zinc in their children's noses and the kids soon lost their sense of smell. Research showed that applying zinc to the olfactory (smell) nerve of a guinea pig destroyed the nerve. The same may occur in humans.

Paradoxically, we sometimes use orally ingested zinc as a treatment for certain forms of loss of the ability to taste, but the direct application of zinc to the nasal apparatus can truly destroy the ability to smell. So, I discourage taking Zicam for a cold because it may cause olfactory damage. Unfortunately, the product falls under the rubric of natural, relatively unregulated remedies, so it remains on the market.

DON'T IGNORE OLD WIVES' TALES

No one has scientifically documented that drinking hot tea, orange juice, or chicken broth actually cures a cold or clears up sinus symptoms. That doesn't mean, however, we should stop doing things that we perceive as taking care of ourselves. Some people feel better wrapped up in a blanket and stretched out on the couch when they have a cold; others need to be in bed with extra covers. Some people begin to crave ginger ale or they drink hot tea only when they're sick. When they're well, neither ginger ale nor hot tea have any appeal at all.

It is likely that the special cravings we have when we're ill are related to a phenomenon known as "olfactory-evoked nostalgia." As the term implies, certain smells will send us into a nostalgic reverie. The scents themselves are not important, but the association with the past is significant. When we studied this phenomenon at the Smell & Taste Treatment and Research Foundation, we found regional and generational differences when it came to the smells that induced nostalgia. For example, older midwesterners identified farm animals and mown grass as their favorite smells of the past, while younger people in general preferred artificial scents such as Play-Doh and Pez candy. By definition, nostalgia is a memory of an idealized past, a time we perceive as simpler and better. A particular smell will send us back to that time, and since we've idealized it, we enjoy the experience.

In all the research we've done at our foundation about favorite smells, we have always found that the odors people like or with which they have positive associations are more likely to make them feel better. A pleasing aroma lifts the spirits. Self-care for colds works the same way. If your mother gave you milk toast when you were sick, then when you get sick as an adult you might crave milk toast. It's part of the nostalgic response. It sounds contradictory, but surrounding yourself with the foods you associate with being taken care of when you were sick as a child may help you feel better as an adult, even though these things may not change the course of your cold.

Common sense tells us that even though these emotional self-care measures haven't been scientifically validated, they usually comfort us in a fundamental way, probably through a nostalgic response. The common cold is one of those annoying realities of life.

To summarize:

1. Colds are caused by viruses and they are a common human malady.

2. Sensible self-care measures, such as consuming extra fluids (especially water) and getting extra rest, are usually all that's required. In addition, avoid iced drinks and smoke from any source (because they interfere with the movement of cilia) and antihistamines (because they dry the mucous membranes in the nose).

3. Many colds last longer than a week or ten days—probably more than 25 percent of colds will linger for two or more weeks.

4. If you have a cold for longer than a week, your chances of being misdiagnosed with a sinus infection increase because, contrary to conventional wisdom, it is relatively rare for a cold to turn into true sinusitis.

Chapter 3

Acute Sinusitis: A Complex Condition

Unfortunately, we must approach any discussion of sinusitis with an understanding that many doctors do not accurately define acute sinusitis and no unified diagnostic procedures or treatments exist, although most practitioners follow general guidelines. This lack of finality of definition and diagnostic procedures leads to a diagnosis that depends on the definition used by the practitioners you consult. For example, if your current difficulties began with acute sinus symptoms following a cold, you probably saw your family doctor. But if your condition became chronic, you may have been referred to an ear, nose, and throat (ENT) specialist, who was likely predisposed to look at your symptoms as sinusitis. If headache is a major symptom, your family doctor may have seen that as a clue and referred you to a neurologist for evaluation. In any case, your chances of resolving your condition are greatest when your doctor or doctors recognize that coexisting conditions are common, not rare.

Some patients see more than one doctor within each specialty because initial treatment may not be effective, the medications stop working, or they are told they need specialized testing for allergies, polyps, or headaches. A variety of tests may be recommended to look closely at the nose and the ears, but the diagnosis is primarily based on symptoms and signs. If treatment appears to work, of course it appears that the diagnosis was correct, despite the fact that the diagnosis was wrong and your symptoms would have resolved on their own, even without any treatment at all!

When it comes to acute sinus infections, the newer, high-tech imaging tests are a mixed blessing—imaging tests can reveal abnormalities in the sinuses that might or might not mean the diagnosis of sinusitis is accurate. Imaging tests have revealed that about 70 percent of the population have visible abnormalities of the sinuses. These abnormalities have little to do with the probability of developing sinusitis and may have nothing to do with current symptoms. In some cases, of course, results of imaging tests combined with a history of chronic symptoms may lead to surgery to remove polyps or to correct anatomical abnormalities. Unfortunately, however, this kind of surgery frequently does not relieve sinusitis-like symptoms.

The beginning of a long journey to find the cure for sinus symptoms often begins with a painful sinus infection (or the diagnosis of one) and for some people may end up in the operating room years later! Fortunately, most people will never need sinus or nasal surgery. Equally important, many people will not need extensive diagnostic tests or drugs.

WHEN A COLD IS NO LONGER A COLD

The last chapter discussed the overlapping symptoms of a common cold caused by a virus, and sinusitis, an infection caused by bacteria. According to conventional wisdom, the signs that a cold (caused by a virus) has turned into a bacterial infection include the following:

- a fever higher than 100 degrees Fahrenheit
- an earache, one or both ears
- tender glands (lymph nodes) in the neck
- worsening cough that produces thick mucus that may be yellow or green
- persistent sore throat
- hoarseness that persists
- worsening malaise and fatigue
- diminished ability to smell and taste
- halitosis
- nasal congestion

In addition, if a cold lingers for more than ten days, a diagnosis of sinus infection may result, even without the addition of the above symptoms. Again, this may depend on your individual physician's guidelines for this illness. The above symptoms may also occur in an acute sinusitis infection that flares up in connection with allergies or asthma. Alternatively, this list of symptoms may also be associated with the flu.

Sinus infections are also classified based on the sinuses affected. For example, maxillary sinusitis indicates an infection in the maxillary sinuses in the middle of the face, on one or both sides. When all the sinuses are involved, the term *pansinusitis* is used.

Unfortunately, as I'll discuss later, facial pain or pressure is often seen as an indicator of sinusitis, even when other symptoms are not present. However, facial pain is a symptom of other conditions, such as migraine headache, which also interferes with the ability to smell and may involve congestion. In addition, it's unclear whether facial pain or headache is a primary symptom of sinusitis. If nasal congestion is present, which is often the case with headache syndromes and other conditions, that symptom alone may lead your doctor to conclude that you have a bacterial sinus infection, or sinusitis. I believe part of the confusion exists because drug advertisers link headaches with the sinuses. Moreover, dental procedures can cause congestion and facial pain, but that does not mean a sinus infection is present. In fact, dental pain may be a symptom of problems that do not involve the teeth or sinuses at all.

POSSIBLE CAUSES OF SINUS SYMPTOMS AND INFECTIONS

Certain underlying conditions and situations may make one more susceptible to sinusitis-like symptoms as well as true sinusitis. As you can see from the following list, these include environmental factors such as high altitude flight to microscopic cellular mechanisms within the body itself.

Flight

In addition to a common cold, sinus symptoms and/or an acute infection can result from changes in air pressure. In susceptible people, flying can cause the ear fullness you experience when the eustachian tube works to equalize pressure changes. This ear popping is a mechanism designed to protect the structures in your head. These pressure changes can make the sinus membranes swell, however; in some cases, this leads to mucus stagnation, creating the conditions for an infection. If you have a cold, taking an OTC decongestant (if they're safe for you) before a flight can keep the nasal passages open and help prevent this stagnation. Short of taking a medication, I recommend chewing a piece of gum because it helps the eustachian tube do its job effectively. Always drink plenty of water before and during a long flight, because drying of the nasal passages promotes stagnation in the river of mucus. Divers also experience changes in air pressure, and susceptible individuals are more likely to develop congestion that may lead to infection.

The Pill

Pregnant women and women taking birth control pills may also experience nasal symptoms. In pregnancy it's known as "rhinitis of pregnancy," and the term also is applied when the hormonal changes induced by the birth control pill mimic the same symptoms. Rhinitis of pregnancy is not a sinus infection; however, over time, the congestion may slow the river of mucus and create the condition for an infection to develop. This is problematic because pregnant women are generally advised not to take medications, even antibiotics, and most doctors do not like to prescribe them except in extreme situations. For the most part, pregnant women are advised to use safe self-care measures, such as saline irrigation (discussed in chapter 9) to keep the "river flowing." The goal is to keep hormonally induced congestion from developing into a sinus infection.

Asthma and Allergies

As previously mentioned, individuals with asthma and/or allergies are considered more at risk for developing sinus infections. Sinus problems, asthma, and allergic responses are often intertwined and will be discussed in detail later. An infection can trigger an asthma attack; polyps are common among those with both asthma and allergies, and polyps slow down mucus flow. The resulting stagnation is the prime setup for a sinus infection. This may appear like a cycle, but it is more like crossing lines with the intersections differing widely among individuals.

Immune Weakness

Immunosuppression, meaning that the immune system does not function normally, or in common terms is "weakened," renders individuals more susceptible to infections of all types. Those undergoing radiation therapy and chemotherapy for cancer are considered immunosuppressed, as are patients who have had organ transplants. HIV-positive patients and those with AIDS also fall into this category. As you can see, this includes many millions of patients every year. Certain types of organisms, such as fungus, also grow in the sinuses of immunosuppressed individuals (and others), complicating both susceptibility and treatment. We'll discuss the issue of fungi later because its link with sinusitis may represent a breakthrough in the theories about sinusitis and hence, effective treatments. Recognition of nasal fungi is part of the "new thinking" in the ENT field and may change approaches to treatment, especially when sinusitis has become chronic.

HOW TO INTERPRET YOUR DOCTOR'S ADVICE

If fever persists, the neck glands stay swollen and tender, and a cough is persistent and violent, a cold is no longer a common cold that will likely run its course. If you have these symptoms and see a doctor only to be told that you have a bacterial sinus infection, I suggest that you do not accept that diagnosis based on the symptoms alone. Based on current knowledge, a sinus puncture is the only sure way to determine if an infection exists. However, this procedure applies only to the maxillary sinuses; the other sinuses are not accessible. To further complicate the diagnostic process, little scientific evidence supports using X rays, CT scans, ultrasound, nasal endoscopy, or nasal swabs to accurately diagnose a sinus infection. (Ultrasound appears to be the least effective of the imaging tests.) This is not the time to become one of the "statistical" subjects who is treated on the basis of national cost-benefit analysis, so I suggest asking more questions before submitting to any treatment.

The idea of having a "sinus puncture" procedure may seem novel to you, and you may wonder why it hasn't been suggested as a diagnostic procedure. In more than twenty years of practicing medicine, I have yet to meet a doctor who performs a sinus puncture to confirm or rule out the presence of a sinus infection (except in emergency situations). Most patients have never even heard of the procedure. The fact is, they are rarely done. Instead, as previously stated, sinusitis is routinely diagnosed on the basis of symptoms and signs, and antibiotics are prescribed.

Unless you have an allergy to penicillin, you will most likely be given a prescription for amoxicillin, generally in either 250- or 500-mg doses taken three times a day for ten days. Children's doses are about half the adult doses. If not amoxicillin, you may be given a folate inhibitor, another class of antibiotics, which includes trimethoprim sulfamethoxazole.

Always take the whole course of treatment, even if you begin to feel better in a few days, which is expected. Some doctors prescribe the antibiotic for fourteen days, with the assumption that this increased dosage will go another mile, so to speak, to prevent recurrence. Amoxicillin or folate inhibitors are generally prescribed whether or not a culture is performed because these two classes of antibiotics are considered effective and safe in most cases. They are also the least expensive antibiotics currently available.

Although there are variations in treatment, if the amoxicillin does not begin to clear up symptoms, you will generally be re-treated with another antibiotic, which could include Bactrim, Septra, Ceclor, or Augmentin. It is possible you will be given one of these instead of amoxicillin in the first place. (If this is the case, be sure to ask why.) Of course, a culture would help determine the antibiotic that is a "match" for specific bacteria, which is why a culture may theoretically shorten treatment time.

Your physician may recommend OTC decongestants containing cough expectorants (mucus thinners) or decongestants with analgesics (pain relievers). Some types are available by prescription only (see the list in the appendix). To be sure that these products are safe for you, make certain your doctor is aware of any underlying condition such as heart disease, hypertension, diabetes, or thyroid disease. If your sleep is interrupted your doctor may suggest a cough suppressant for nighttime use.

Antihistamines are not generally recommended because they tend to dry the sinuses and this thickens the mucus and prevents the cilia from pushing the river of mucus through and out of the sinuses. The sluggish mucus flow may set up the condition for reinfection. If you decide to use OTC nasal sprays, remember that they can be addictive, so limit their use to no more than two or three days.

WAITING IT OUT

The way sinusitis is generally explained, cold symptoms that last more than ten days or two weeks indicate that a bacterial infection has developed. However, about 25 percent of cases of viral rhinitis (the common cold) last longer than two weeks. By one calculation, Americans have a total of about one *billion* colds a year; if one quarter of them last more than two weeks, that's about 250 million "atypical" colds. Since sinusitis often is misdiagnosed, this results in unnecessary antibiotic treatment and perhaps delayed treatment for the true cause of the symptoms. Unfortunately, the problem is deeper and more complex than that.

It may sound shocking or discouraging to state that in most cases, "doing nothing" and "doing something" result in about the same treatment results. However, in one clinical trial that included patients diagnosed with acute bacterial sinusitis, 85 percent of patients improved (1) from doing nothing or (2) from taking a placebo (an inactive substance). In fact, the highest cure rate in the study was seen in the group taking the placebo! It's important that these patients were diagnosed using signs and symptoms only. No other diagnostic tests were performed as further documentation. This situation actually mimics clinical practice. In addition, the recurrence rate was lower among patients taking the placebo than among those in the antibiotic group.

Another study, reported in JAMA (*Journal of the American Medical Association*), looked at treatment for 3,038 patients who had reported sinus headaches and were diagnosed with sinusitis and treated with antibiotics. The study concluded that only 8 (0.3 percent) individuals in this group actually had a sinus infection! The article raised the obvious concern that this kind of misdiagnosis contributes to the creation of bacterial resistance. Although I will discuss the whole issue of sinus headaches in chapter 6, it is important to realize that experiencing facial pain, even around the eyes and cheeks, does not necessarily mean that you have a sinus headache. Beyond that, pain in the region of the sinuses does not point to an infection.

Overall, a review of literature dealing with sinusitis treatment concludes that in most cases "watchful waiting" is probably the best course when an acute bacterial sinus infection appears the most likely diagnosis. By the way, I am not recommending that you avoid seeing your doctor. In rare situations, a sinus infection can develop into a serious, even life-threatening situation that involves loss of vision or a brain abscess. These occur in about 1 in 95,000 cases, and your doctor can monitor unusual or changing symptoms, such as swelling around the eyes and visual disturbance. Most doctors never see one of these complications. In more than twenty years of practice, I've seen only one such complication resulting from an acute bacterial sinus infection.

After looking at study after study, and numerous articles that review all the literature about acute bacterial sinusitis, certain realities emerge:

1. Acute bacterial sinusitis is diagnosed based on signs and symptoms (which may or may not lead to an accurate diagnosis).
2. Treatment follows the fairly standard path of recommending antibiotics.
3. When antibiotics are worthwhile for acute sinusitis, amoxicillin and folate inhibitors are as effective as the newer, more expensive broad-spectrum antibiotics.
4. The OTC cold remedies that contain decongestants and

the OTC nasal sprays do not appear to affect the severity or duration of a sinus infection.

5. The vast majority of diagnosed sinus infections will resolve on their own in ten days to two weeks.

6. It appears that many diagnosed sinus infections are actually "bad" colds, meaning that the symptoms increase and decrease in severity and make life miserable until they finally resolve after a period of time that may stretch to four weeks. I calculate this based on the idea that most adults will not seek medical care for what they perceive is a cold unless it doesn't clear up in ten days to two weeks. At that point, they may take an antibiotic or do nothing, and most of the time, no matter which path they take, their symptoms will clear up in another ten days to two weeks. Even if these infections are not "bad colds," and truly are bacterial infections, it appears the majority resolve on their own anyway.

7. Unless there is a demonstrated reason why "watchful waiting" is unwise in your case, it is probably the most sensible path.

8. Before you reach any conclusions about the right diagnosis in your case, especially if you have recurrent sinus infections, it is important to investigate information about headaches and allergies.

SELF-CARE HELPS THE SYMPTOMS, BUT NOT THE DISEASE

Based on the medical literature, typical self-care measures do not appear to influence the resolution of a sinus infection or a cold. Of course, it makes sense to drink fluids, rest and relax at home, try to sleep more than usual, avoid exposure to common pollutants such as cigarette smoke, and use a humidifier and/or steam inhalation. I discuss sinus irrigation elsewhere and it appears that it's becoming increasingly popular as a self-care measure for both prevention and treatment. However, like most OTC therapies and even the most standard self-care techniques, it hasn't been adequately studied and no one can definitively say that any of these home remedies shorten the length of a cold. Still, as I said previously, if you feel better and are comforted by certain foods or by wrapping up in a favorite blanket, by all means go for comfort.

If you have sinusitis-like symptoms, and you use common-sense self-care measures, your symptoms should clear up in approximately two weeks. In general, these sinus symptoms do not pose a great risk but are annoying, even debilitating while they last. Once they clear up, life goes back to normal. However, some individuals find that sinus infection–like symptoms either start a cycle or are part of a cycle in which bouts with these sinus symptoms seem to pile up. Unfortunately, for some this situation may last for years. And as I said, the road to surgery often starts with a cold that docsn't go away in a couple of weeks. (The next chapter discusses what happens when sinusitis-like symptoms appear to evolve into a chronic condition.)

WHY YOU *MUST* MONITOR YOUR SYMPTOMS

A true sinus infection is a medical emergency and potentially serious, which is why it is critical that you monitor your symptoms. One of the reasons some doctors generally recommend antibiotics to treat sinusitis-like symptoms is because the complications of a true sinus infection can be so serious. These complications can involve the eye (orbital) or the brain (intracranial). CT scans can detect complications involving bony tissue, such as orbital cellulitis or abscess or mucoceles (mucus-filled cysts). MRI is better at investigating soft tissue inflammation, such as what is present in brain abscesses and meningitis. Eye complications may produce symptoms such as swelling and redness around the eyes, bulging or drooping eyelids, eye pain, blurred vision, and other symptoms associated with vision.

These complications are medical emergencies and require hospitalization and IV antibiotics. Fortunately, such complications are very rare and the possibility they will develop does not warrant prescribing antibiotics for every case of sinusitis-like symptoms, especially since the symptoms are likely caused by another condition in the first place.

SUMMING UP

Because true sinusitis is a serious infection and usually occurs in individuals who are immunocompromised because of another condition (e.g., chemotherapy, unstable diabetes, AIDS), sinusitis-like symptoms are often overtreated. Remember:

1. Studies have shown that antibiotic treatment is routinely recommended for colds that last longer than a week or ten days because it is presumed that a sinus infection has developed.
2. No specific tests are generally performed to confirm the actual presence of an infection and diagnosis is made on the basis of signs and symptoms.
3. Current research suggests that most sinusitis-like symptoms resolve in ten days to two weeks on their own, making the concept of "watchful waiting" a sensible way to handle lingering cold and sinusitis-like symptoms.

Chapter 4

Chronic Sinusitis: When Symptoms Go On and On . . .

In 1982, the National Center for Health Statistics put the number of *chronic* sinusitis sufferers at twenty-seven million cases, but by 1993, it had jumped to thirty-seven million, which is about one in seven of us (and the number continues to grow). In addition, according to the literature, these thirty-seven million men and women in the United States describe sinusitis as a *major* health problem.

Just to be clear about definitions, a chronic problem simply means that it is firmly established, long lasting, persistent, and unfortunately, often intractable. Without being flip, it's no exaggeration to say that chronic sinusitis-like symptoms are more than a disease, they become a "lifestyle." The lost work hours cause an economic impact, medical costs mount, family life suffers, and the problem cuts into all leisure activities. Of course, as I've mentioned, I believe it is likely that many millions of these individuals actually have migraine headaches, or another condition, because sinusitis, both acute and chronic, is so often misdiagnosed. But no matter how we label or divide the numbers, we are talking about a serious health problem—we could call it a crisis. And while sinusitis is rarely fatal, patients routinely tell their doctors that at least on some days, it's difficult to put in the effort to live a full life.

These growing numbers also mean that chronic sinusitis has now become the most common long-term medical condition in the country, more pervasive than asthma, arthritis, hypertension, and back pain. (Back pain was always considered the leading cause of lost productivity and missed workdays, but it appears that sinusitis now has that dubious distinction.) When sinusitis becomes a chronic problem, low energy is a major complaint, so it is no wonder that every aspect of life is affected.

The Centers for Disease Control (CDC) report that the group of typical sinus symptoms account for twelve million doctor visits annually, and the success rate of any treatment for the diagnosis (usually sinusitis) is *subjectively* measured. This means that patients report how they feel without any objective measures, such as radiological tests, that show the presence or absence of abnormalities. Some people believe that sinusitis can be demonstrated with CT or MRI scans that show thickening of the walls (epithelial thickening). However, this thickening is often seen in those with sinus symptoms and those without any sinus complaints at all. Furthermore, the thickening within the sinus walls may not change after a full course of antibiotics. Because we do not yet know that epithelial thickening is an abnormal finding in all individuals, the usefulness of CT or MRI scans is limited as diagnostic or objective tools to assess the success of treatment. Thus, treatment is very challenging because it is difficult to determine if symptom relief can be attributed to treatment or the placebo effect; this also makes reliable data concerning the true success rates for treatment, including surgery, problematic.

A Harvard study released in 1990 claimed the total annual drug cost in the United States to treat sinusitis was *$45 billion*, of which $15 billion was spent on OTC decongestants, nasal sprays, and so forth. Today, hundreds of millions of dollars are spent marketing sinus medications to both physicians and consumers, and at the annual per-patient cost for drugs of $1,220, this is an expensive chronic condition—before we even begin to look at the annual cost of surgery (see chapter 10).

DIAGNOSTIC DEFINITIONS

Diagnostic labels for sinusitis are based on broad definitions and are useful when we try to gather and compare treatment data. However, they may or may not be relevant in your individual case. Although the definitions vary somewhat, chronic sinusitis is described as:

- sinus symptoms that last longer than eight to twelve weeks;
- three to four recurrent infections in a period of six months to a year.

Sometimes sinusitis symptoms that last longer than four weeks, but less than twelve weeks, are called *subacute sinusitis*. Another type of chronic sinusitis is defined as chronic inflammation of the mucous membranes and some nasal secretions, but often without signs of a bacterial infection or cold symptoms. These individuals may have some nasal symptoms, but in general they do not feel ill. It is not known how many, or for that matter, *if any* of these patients actually suffer from true sinusitis!

WHAT CHRONIC SINUSITIS IS *NOT*

One of the biggest challenges we face when treating sinusitis is that it's confused with other conditions (see below). For example, chronic sinusitis is not allergic rhinitis, though the two are often confused, and having one condition doesn't preclude the other. The same is true for asthma. In addition, nasal congestion that occurs with migraine headache is not sinusitis. Chronic sinusitis *may* include olfactory loss, but you can't conclude that you have chronic sinusitis if your ability to smell is impaired, although paradoxically, in some cases, smell loss is the *only* symptom of chronic sinusitis.

Here are some other causes of congestion that could lead to a label of chronic sinusitis:

- Even though hypertension does not cause nasal blockage, medications used to treat it can cause nasal stuffiness (and sometimes a dry cough). Since millions of people use these medications, often changing from one to another, and with dosages varying and changing, this may be an underrecognized origin of chronic congestion.
- The upper teeth border on the maxillary sinuses, so an abscess or other dental condition can affect them, perhaps even causing congestion. In fact, if nasal symptoms, such as congestion, suddenly flare up when you have no history of any sinus problems, consider a visit to the dentist.
- Sinusitis is not the congestion that some women experience during ovulation and pregnancy, or that some women endure on oral contraceptives. The hormonal changes that occur during pregnancy cause swelling in the nasal membranes, resulting in congestion. The swelling causes little "tornadoes" in the nose, often enhancing the

ability to smell. During ovulation women have a better sense of smell than during any other time in the cycle. Some pregnant women may find the swelling and congestion bothersome and they believe they have a nagging cold or perhaps have developed an allergy with pregnancy and at ovulation. The mucus tends to be thin and clear, as it is in allergic rhinitis. I do not recommend using nasal sprays or taking decongestants during pregnancy because the effects of such medication on the fetus are unknown.

This nasal congestion may be a natural state in pregnancy and during ovulation, but may be confused with sinusitis. In addition, women on birth control pills may think the congestion is a symptom of chronic sinusitis, especially if they have a history of sinus symptoms. Because normal menstrual and pregnancy congestion symptoms can easily be misdiagnosed, virtually every woman could be misdiagnosed as having sinusitis at some point in her life.

• Remember, too, that both sexes experience nasal congestion during sexual arousal. This, too, is a natural response, and may be part of the olfactory mechanism that allows us to detect pheromones. When the nose is partially stuffed, inhalation induces little eddy currents, or "tornadoes," to develop in the nose, causing more odorant to reach the olfactory epithelium than when there is no stuffiness. In other words, the sense of smell improves with mild congestion.

WORKING DEFINITIONS

Chronic sinusitis symptoms cover considerable ground and may or may not coexist with other problems. Indeed, to list symptoms of sinusitis means listing symptoms involved in other conditions, because they can overlap to a large degree. The following are a few of the commonly reported symptoms among patients who receive a diagnosis of chronic sinusitis:

- almost permanent congestion, only temporarily relieved
- runny nose/thick discharge
- persistent ear fullness
- smell loss
- mouth breathing/sleep disturbance
- dental pain
- throat and voice symptoms
- fatigue/run-down feeling
- irritability
- sense of debilitation or as if living with a "disability"
- headaches/facial pain

Clearly, these symptoms can be linked to other conditions, which may coexist with sinusitis and be related to it, or they may be signs of an unrelated condition. It is also possible that the asthma, allergies, and sinusitis are interacting conditions: the postnasal drip from sinusitis makes asthma worse and then the allergies exacerbate the asthma attack caused by the postnasal drip.

In general, stubborn or recurring sinus infections are commonly treated with antibiotics, which usually involves repeating treatment or using different antibiotics until some relief occurs. Sometimes, long-term, in-home intravenous antibiotics may be recommended when the physician believes that extended antibiotic treatment may clear up a chronic infection. In addition to antibiotics, the physician may prescribe steroid nasal sprays.

Prior to agreeing to surgery, I recommend that sinusitis patients, including children, have tests that measure immune system function. This means looking beyond the fact that an infection is present and then establishing the particular bacteria. These tests evaluate why the person is susceptible. For example, one study showed that 30 percent of participants had immune system abnormalities. I advocate assuming that incidence of an immune function problem is high among individuals who have numerous recurrent infections. When an elderly person breaks a bone, a physician doesn't just treat the break but looks for the reasons why the person fell and the bone broke. The physician rules out neurological problems that might cause unstable gait and tests for osteoporosis. By the same token, shouldn't time be spent trying to discover why a person is vulnerable to chronic sinusitis?

NASAL POLYPS

Nasal polyps are not always present with chronic sinusitis, but they're often a coexisting condition. Polyps can occur anywhere in the body, and in the nose they are grape-like growths inside the nasal passages. They may be caused by sensitivity to aspirin or by allergies, although the reasons they form are not well understood. Polyps may form when the mucous membrane grows excessively, as often occurs with allergies. Their presence then narrows the nasal passages or forms small barriers that slow down or block normal mucus flow, which then indirectly causes congestion and perhaps sinusitis. Polyps may also impair the sense of smell. While not a direct component of asthma, polyps are common among asthmatics.

If you have polyps, nonsurgical treatment usually involves taking an antibiotic (because the stagnant pond created in the sinuses is a perfect environment for bacteria to breed) and steroid medication, which acts on the polyps and shrinks them. Your doctor may suggest a repeated antibiotic treatment and may add a steroid nasal spray. This combination treatment may be recommended for chronic sinus infections, too. Polyp tissue may be removed surgically, but unfortunately, they often return.

If polyps develop, or the sinuses remain "cloudy," or the symptoms of infection persist, then surgery is often recommended. I'll examine surgical options in chapter 10, but the following discussion should clarify some conditions that are commonly mistaken for chronic sinusitis.

CAN REFLUX DISEASE AND SINUSITIS BE CONFUSED?

Gastroesophageal reflux disease, commonly called GERD, is currently linked with chronic sinusitis. It may be a cause of chronic congestion and other symptoms, or on the other hand, it may be confused with chronic sinusitis. GERD develops because the valve between the esophagus and the stomach does not work properly, which allows the stomach acids to travel up through the esophagus and cause a variety of symptoms, including heartburn and thick phlegm that can lead to inflammation of the esophagus. Symptoms are usually worse in the morning, because the "backup" of the stomach acid generally occurs at night.

Individuals with GERD experience the following symptoms, most often in the morning:

- sore or burning throat or a tickling in the throat
- bad breath or a sour or bitter taste in the mouth

- hoarseness and problems with the voice
- a chronic cough, the need to clear the throat, or a lump in the throat
- regurgitating food and liquids
- burning or raw mouth or tongue

As you can see, along with the presence of thick mucus, the other respiratory symptoms can lead to misdiagnosis. In addition, GERD can make asthma a more complicated disease to control because theophylline (a bronchodilator medication) may affect the action of the valve between the esophagus and the stomach.

It is entirely possible to be unaware of GERD, especially if you have a history of sinus or respiratory disease. A variety of tests can establish GERD and a combination of medication and lifestyle changes can ease symptoms. I recommend investigating the possibility that GERD is either responsible for symptoms that mimic sinusitis or is playing a role in exacerbating the cycle of respiratory symptoms that persist in those who have been diagnosed with chronic sinusitis and regularly seek help for it.

ASTHMA OR SINUSITIS—OR BOTH

Sinusitis is not asthma, but up to 80 percent of people with asthma experience nasal symptoms. This raises the question, are those symptoms due to sinusitis or does sinusitis *induce* asthma? When you try to put together the pieces of the puzzle that represents your symptoms, consider the possibility that chronic sinusitis has been misdiagnosed and may be asthma. Nasal congestion is often part of the asthma attack, which may mean that treating the asthma can help the sinus symptoms.

Asthma is a specific disease, with specific triggers. Many asthma sufferers have their first asthma attack in childhood, but the disease can appear at any age. In addition, a family history of asthma increases your chances of developing the disease.

An asthma attack involves:

- spasms and inflammation in the airways, which are triggered by allergens, certain kinds of activities, and cold air
- swelling of the mucous membranes that line the bronchi
- excessive mucus production
- spasms in the bronchial muscles (bronchospasm)

These symptoms or "actions" contribute to a narrowing of the airways, which:

- makes it difficult to breathe
- produces wheezing and shortness of breath
- brings on a cough with thickening mucus
- often results in a tightening in the chest

Anything that causes airway inflammation and bronchospasm can trigger asthma. Allergens are a major trigger, but activities such as exercise, singing, crying, or even laughing can bring on symptoms. The severity of attacks may vary, but asthma is always a serious issue because it can be life threatening. Unfortunately, chest X rays do not necessarily reveal any abnormality. Since you breathe normally during a routine office visit, your doctor often can't diagnose asthma based on observed respiratory symptoms, so pulmonary function tests are necessary. Sinus symptoms and nasal polyps may be part of the picture. The postnasal drip that causes a cough can then be an indirect trigger for an asthma attack.

Asthma is treated in numerous ways. Oral steroids may be given to reverse a severe attack and inhaled steroids are used for a milder attack. Those with asthma probably have a bronchodilator, most likely an inhaler, which allows the airways to open and helps restore normal breathing. Thus, even though asthma and sinusitis are not the same disease, it appears they often occur together, and about 80 percent of asthmatics have nasal symptoms.

About ten million Americans have asthma and a 42 percent increase occurred between 1982 and 1992. Worldwide, the rising asthma rates remain a mystery, particularly the childhood asthma rate, which doubled between 1975 and 1995. The finger of blame for this rise (among adults and children) usually points to the spread of global industrialization, with the accompanying increase in air pollution. On the face of it, the link seems logical, but studies that have attempted to document that link do not show the expected results. In the 1990s, a study compared asthma rates among 5,600 children in Dresden, a polluted city located in the former East Germany, and Munich, a city located in West Germany that is noted for its clean air. Asthma rates were higher in Munich than in Dresden, which was an unexpected result.

Demographic studies often document changes in disease rates among populations that relocate. For example, when individuals moved from a particular Polynesian island to New Zealand (a country known for clean air), they doubled their risk of developing asthma. Demographic studies have also shown the same trend among those who move from the Philippines to the United States and for those who move from Asia and East Africa to England. Interestingly, several decades ago the Chinese of Taiwan began to adopt a more Westernized lifestyle, and now asthma rates among children went up *eight* times since the mid-1970s. Asthma is higher in the urban, wealthier areas of Ghana than in the poorer rural villages. On the other hand, asthma risk is the same in Brazil and Peru among the rich and the poor. Therefore, even though pollution, which is part of the "affluence" that comes along with industrialization, is often said to be responsible for rising rates of asthma, the research doesn't substantiate this belief. We can probably say that air pollution may exacerbate asthma in some cases, and it may cause a small number of cases to develop, although we can't yet quantify that. Although we still do not know why asthma is on the rise, it is probably not coincidental that chronic sinusitis rates also have risen.

SUMMARY

1. No absolute definition of chronic sinusitis exists, but the condition is defined as either persistent symptoms or frequently recurring symptoms.
2. Persistent nasal congestion and related symptoms have many causes, so do not assume that you have chronic sinus disease. Look for other causes before accepting a "label" of chronic sinusitis.
3. I suggest investigating the possibility that dental problems, GERD, nasal polyps, or asthma are causing your symptoms.

Chapter 5

Allergies Versus Sinusitis

Chronic sinusitis can easily be confused with allergies, and almost 60 percent of patients seen for sinusitis have allergic rhinitis. Some OTC allergy medications sometimes relieve sinus symptoms and that leaves the impression that *allergies* and *chronic sinus symptoms* are interchangeable terms for conditions that are nearly identical—at least in terms in how they "look" and feel. But the thin, watery mucus generally triggered by allergies is one clue that sinusitis is not the root cause of a group of similar symptoms. In addition, seasonal allergies provide another clue that the symptoms are linked to external substances that cause a flare-up that goes away once the season changes. The symptoms of chronic sinusitis do not follow a predictable pattern. On the other hand, allergies can contribute to the development of sinus infections.

THE RELATIONSHIP BETWEEN ALLERGIC RHINITIS AND SINUSITIS

It's well documented that allergic rhinitis and sinusitis often "hang out" together. Although comparative X-ray studies may not tell the whole story, one study showed that 53 percent of children with allergic rhinitis had abnormal sinus X rays; another study reported that up to 70 percent of children with allergy and chronic rhinitis had abnormal findings on sinus X rays. Many studies show a high percentage of people with both allergic rhinitis and sinusitis. The only caution here is that *these numbers may not be strictly accurate because the individuals may or may not have had true sinusitis.* It isn't surprising that diseases that result from a sluggish river of mucus tend to be linked, however, and even difficult to differentiate. Viral rhinitis, the common cold, also occurs in the spring and fall and many people may have allergies they interpret as "just a cold." It's also possible that a cold can be labeled an allergy, which may then add that label to either a person's official or "self-diagnosed" medical history.

What we can conclude is that allergic rhinitis doesn't directly cause sinusitis, but it is a risk factor in eventual development of chronic sinusitis. Therefore, it is wise to diagnose and treat allergies as a preventive measure, because chronic sinusitis is even more problematic than living with allergies.

About 20 percent of adults and children have seasonal or perennial allergic rhinitis. Allergies may also be a cause of a certain type of viral ear infection, OME (otitis media with effusion). This type of ear infection can involve nasal inflammation and obstruction caused by nasal allergy, viral infection, or both. Upper respiratory tract infection (URI) occurring in patients with nasal allergies may have enhanced inflammatory responses in the nose and eustachian tube that then lead to obstruction and OME.

Simply defined, allergies involve being hypersensitive to a substance (allergen) that then causes a response in the body that produces symptoms. (The word *allergy* actually derives from the Greek words for "other action.") The response to a foreign "invader" is an immune system function, so when a sensitive person comes in contact with an allergen, the immune system responds by producing antibodies.

The immune system is supposed to be vigilant in protecting the body; it produces specific cells to counteract the invaders. For example, we have lymphocytes—white blood cells—that produce plasma cells. The plasma cells then produce antibodies whose job it is to neutralize antigens, a collective term for these invaders. T cells are important for fighting off bacterial and viral infections. B cells are made up of special kinds of proteins called immunoglobulins (Igs). Although there are five different types of Igs, the one called IgE is most involved with allergies. The immune system has a long and efficient memory, so when the body encounters an invading substance it is programmed to recognize it from previous encounters and can immediately deal with it.

Having an allergic response to pollen, for example, can be described as an "overreaction." Pollen is not a harmful substance, but in some people, the body misreads it and sets off an allergic response. This is why some people are allergic to certain plants or foods or naturally occurring substances such as wool or cat dander and others have no reaction at all. When a person with allergies comes in contact with the perceived dangerous substance, the allergen does one of the following:

1. Reacts with IgE on the surface of a type of white blood cell called *basophils*.
2. Reacts with mast cells, which line the GI tract, the skin, and most significant to our discussion, the respiratory tract.

This causes a host of chemical reactions within the basophils or mast cells, including the production and release of histamine, which produces the symptoms we associate with allergies:

- nasal stuffiness and sneezing
- thin, clear nasal mucus
- dry cough
- watery or itchy eyes
- rings or dark circles around the eyes (allergic shiner)
- itchy skin
- a run-down, tired feeling and irritability

Depending on the type of allergy, other physiological responses are possible as well, from headaches to GI symptoms such as heartburn and cramping. Skin conditions such as eczema are also common. Histamine is capable of producing everything from hives to an itching sensation on the roof of the mouth.

Sometimes people confuse the symptoms and label them as sinus infection. However, a true sinus infection is more likely to produce the following:

- a *thick* nasal discharge, not thin discharge
- a *productive* cough, not dry cough

It is necessary to keep the differentiation of symptoms in mind because admittedly they are easy to confuse and overlap in many cases, and allergies can lead to sinus infections.

WHEN ALLERGIC RESPONSES ARE LIFE THREATENING

Any discussion of allergies would be incomplete without a warning about *anaphylactic shock*. Although not specifically related to sinusitis, it is a special situation related to allergies. The term refers to a rare occurrence in which the entire respiratory and circulatory systems react: air passages narrow and blood vessels dilate, making breathing difficult and slowing the pulse. It can cause unconsciousness and in rare situations, death. Unfortunately, we don't necessarily know what we are sensitive to until we come into contact with the potentially fatal invader. For example, an insect sting may cause anaphylactic shock in a very small number of individuals, and since being stung by bees or wasps is not an everyday event, many of us will never know if we are vulnerable to anaphylaxis. Certain foods such as peanuts and shellfish can cause anaphylaxis, as can certain drugs, which is why you are asked if you have any known drug allergies before being given a prescription.

Becoming anaphylactic is a true medical emergency and must be quickly treated with epinephrine. I once reviewed the medical records of a man who was allergic to seafood and began showing symptoms while eating a salad in a seafood restaurant. As it turned out, a patron at a table next to him ordered sizzling shrimp. The cloud of shrimp allergen wafted over to him, and he developed an allergic anaphylactic reaction, his throat closed off, and he died. In 2003, the *Mayo Clinic Proceedings* reported an incident in which a twenty-year-old woman kissed her boyfriend less than an hour after he had eaten shrimp. Her anaphylactic reaction was near fatal, but fortunately, she was taken to the emergency room and treated immediately. In another situation, one of the crew working on trees in my backyard was stung by a hornet from a nest hidden near the top of the tree. I happened to be watching the worker from my window and saw the man descending the tree very quickly, so quickly, in fact, that I thought he was falling and I went out to tend to him. By the time I got there, he was sweating, had difficulty breathing, and his blood pressure had dropped—all symptoms of anaphylactic shock. I called an ambulance and considered doing an emergency tracheotomy, a procedure that opens up an airway through the trachea that allows air into the larynx through a makeshift tube. Because I was at home, my tube would have been a straw and my scalpel a kitchen knife, so I was relieved when the ambulance arrived quickly and treated him immediately with epinephrine.

CAUSES OF ALLERGIES

Allergies are a major cause of respiratory and nasal symptoms. Therefore, it is critical that you find out if you have allergies that are causing either persistent or recurring symptoms. The term *allergic rhinitis* applies to nasal symptoms, and seasonal allergic rhinitis affects about twenty-three million Americans, who respond to specific allergens such as airborne pollens from weeds, spores, molds, and grasses. (According to an article published in JAMA, the incidence of allergic disease has increased substantially from 1980 to 2000.) Furthermore, symptoms caused by the antibodies can resemble sinusitis—runny nose; congestion; sneezing; itching, red, watery eyes; sore throat, and so forth. Ragweed is one of the most common allergens in the United States; it is responsible for much of "autumn allergic misery." Conversely, reaction to grass pollen is responsible for much "spring misery."

Many individuals are allergic to certain foods (e.g., milk,

wheat, shellfish, eggs, pork, and nuts). Virtually any substance may be an allergen, but the following are some of the common categories that produce *respiratory* symptoms:

- dust
- wool and feathers
- pollen
- molds
- smoke (particularly tobacco smoke)
- animals
- various foods

Dust is one of the most common perennial allergies, and is difficult to label, because a dust-free environment is virtually impossible to find. If you suspect an allergy to dust or other common household materials, remove feather pillows or down-filled comforters, wool blankets, and so forth, then remove dust catchers like heavy drapes, books, and rugs and see if the symptoms subside. You can try this for your children as well. I say this because many people have mild allergies to a variety of materials and substances, but do not necessarily need diagnostic tests or treatment. Simply eliminating some of the common "offenders" may narrow down the allergen.

Mold grows in fabric, such as in stuffed furniture stored in the basement where it's cold and damp. Your child's stuffed animals may be a breeding ground for mold, so make sure to keep them clean and dry. Dead vegetation breeds mold as well. If you use a humidifier or vaporizer, keep it cleaned and dry to avoid mold growth. Anytime you see the telltale signs of mildew on old canvas or on damp wood, you know mold spores are breeding.

You may be able to avoid being overwhelmed by pollen if

you don't work in the garden or cut grass. If necessary, stay inside, and if you plan a trip out of town, head to the high mountains or the seashore, where less pollen is found. Some people may be very sensitive to flowers and must avoid having them around, even in an outside garden.

Few people like to hear that "Snowball" and "Fido" are walking allergens. I sure loved the cat (named "Kitty") I had as a child, but I had constant congestion and what I now realize were sinusitis-like symptoms that probably were allergic reactions to my beloved cat. The fact is, we can trace a case of chronic *pseudo*-sinusitis through pet dander. Here's how:

- The pet generates dander.
- The devoted owners—children or adults—are in contact with the allergen.
- The immune response is triggered; IgE is produced.
- Histamine is released.
- Sneezing, runny nose, etc. begins.
- The mucous membrane in the nose swells.
- The flow of the river of mucus slows down.
- Stagnant ponds form in the sinuses.
- Bacteria, viruses, and fungi breed.
- Antihistamine medications dry the sinuses.
- The ostia become blocked.
- Sinusitis-like symptoms begin; they may be confused with the initial response to histamine.
- Ten days later, a bacterial infection is diagnosed.
- Antibiotics seem to clear up the worst of the symptoms, but congestion lingers . . . and the whole cycle repeats.

We could continue here with a sad tale of recurrent symptoms and so forth, but you get the point. It sounds hard hearted, but if you (or your child) have allergies to pets, a cycle can easily begin with an allergic response, but quite literally end up in an operating room because of intractable chronic sinus symptoms. If asthma is involved, a bronchodilator becomes a constant companion, and the respiratory symptoms further become a familiar cyclical pattern. You must decide if having a pet is worth the risk of troublesome allergies and respiratory symptoms. Even shorthaired pets cause allergic reactions, because hair is not the source of dander, the constantly shedding skin is. And birds are not really a solution because they act as allergens to many people as well. Your safest bet may be an aquarium filled with fish.

In recent years, a trend has developed that involves importing various animals—so-called exotic pets. Periodically, we also hear about infectious diseases that can be traced back to them (e.g., "monkey pox," traced to prairie dogs). I do not believe it's wise to introduce these animals into a household when any family member has known allergies to animals or has any respiratory or sinus symptoms. Many arguments exist for avoiding contact with any of these imported animals, but anyone who has asthma, allergies, sinus symptoms, frequent colds, or other respiratory diseases should be especially vigilant.

TESTING FOR AND TREATING ALLERGIES

The two most reliable ways to test for allergies are skin testing and a procedure called radioallergosorbent test (RAST). Skin testing involves using a prick, scratch, or injection to expose the skin (on the back or the arms) to a potential allergen. A positive response means that the skin turned red or swelled. A negative outcome means the skin did not react to the allergen.

These are neither pleasant nor easy tests, particularly for children, and they are time consuming.

RAST involves identifying the antibody proteins produced during an allergic response. RAST is "high tech" compared with skin testing and involves using a blood sample that is tested for its response to allergens. In other words, you don't have to be present and exposed to the allergens yourself. You let your blood tell the tale.

A nasal smear may help establish if nasal symptoms are caused by allergies. During an allergic response *eosinophils*—a type of white blood cell—are produced and can be found in the nasal secretions. The presence of these substances does not tell you what you're allergic to, but rather, provides an additional diagnostic clue.

Food allergies are often diagnosed by eliminating the common foods to which people have allergies, recording all foods eaten, along with the quantities, and then observing and recording symptoms or the lack thereof. "Offending" foods are then reintroduced and the reactions are observed. This is an easy way to identify the most common food allergies, but talk to your doctor about this first.

Seasonal allergies are generally treated with antihistamines (many of which are OTC products). However, do not use OTC allergy medications without discussing the whole picture with your doctor. If you have chronic sinus conditions, these medications may make your situation worse, blocking the symptoms that result from the histamines the body produces. Although a complete list appears in the appendix, both Benadryl and Chlor-Trimeton are examples of popular antihistamines. These medications can make one drowsy, so don't use them if you plan to drive or operate machinery. (Less frequently reported symptoms include blurred vision, nausea, and mental fogginess.) By relieving the runny nose and watery eyes, antihistamines also dry the nose and throat, which may thicken the mucus and create the conditions for bacteria to grow in the stagnant "pond" in the sinuses. More recently, antihistamines designed to avoid the drowsiness have been developed. These are called "non-sedating" allergy medications and include Claritin (OTC) and Zyrtec, Allegra, and Clarinex, which are still available by prescription only.

Astelin is a prescription nasal antihistamine spray (non-steroid). It works quickly and because it isn't taken orally, it doesn't cause drowsiness or many other side effects caused by the oral antihistamines. Flonase spray (a steroid medication, by prescription) acts as an anti-inflammatory and is used either for seasonal allergies or year-round. Similarly, Rhinocort (prescription) is an inhaler used to relieve hay fever symptoms and other causes of nasal inflammation. These medications may interact with other allergy medications, so always ask your doctor about their safe use.

Antihistamine–decongestant combination medications are also available, but remember that those with hypertension or any cardiovascular problems should not use them. Common OTC brands include Allerest, Triaminic, and Claritin D.

Prescription-only steroid medications such as Prednisone and Medrol, both cortisone drugs, decrease inflammation, but because they are powerful substances with potentially serious side effects (water retention, elevated blood pressure, personality changes, insomnia) your doctor will prescribe them for limited use and for severe allergy flare-ups. Nasal steroids, such as Beconase or Flonase, reduce swelling of the nasal membrane. They are less dangerous than oral steroid medications because they do not enter the bloodstream, but they may cause side effects such as nasal irritation and nosebleeds because of their drying effects.

Nasalcrom is the trade name for an OTC (nonsteroid) nasal spray called *intranasal cromolyn sodium*. It has been studied as both a treatment and a preventive, and both decreases inflammation and prevents it when used prophylactically. Nasalcrom is discussed in the literature as valuable precisely because allergic rhinitis so frequently coexists with other conditions—like asthma, ear infections, and sinusitis. And as we've seen, anything you can do to prevent one condition from leading to another is worthwhile.

Intranasal cromolyn sodium is a spray derived from the plant *amni visnaga* and works to inhibit the degranulation of mast cells and the release of the substances that trigger inflammation and the early allergic reactions. This medication acts on eosinophils as well as mast cells. This is interesting because new thinking in the field of chronic sinusitis suggests that eosinophils may be the key to chronic sinusitis. Therefore, if intranasal cromolyn sodium medication can inhibit eosinophils, it may work to prevent sinusitis. Theoretically, this would work over half the time, given that over half the patients who believe they have sinusitis have allergic rhinitis. Consider asking your doctor about intranasal cromolyn sodium.

According to the literature reviews, intranasal cromolyn sodium has several advantages over other allergy medications:

- It does not have a sedating effect and, therefore, does not have an adverse effect on productivity and is safe at work and at school.
- It is safe for individuals, including many older persons, who are taking medications for hypertension, diabetes, seizure disorders, and prostate disease.

- Individuals who do not like using any OTC or prescription drugs often find it acceptable because of its lack of side effects.
- Athletes who are routinely tested for drug use may not be able to use OTC allergy medications, but intranasal cromolyn sodium is acceptable.
- It can be used prior to exposure to a known allergen, thereby preventing an allergy attack, so it is useful for campers and or for any outdoor activity, or when you know you'll be visiting a home with furry pets.
- Unlike steroid drugs, this drug does not affect bone mineral density.

Although it appears to be safe during pregnancy, *pregnant women should talk with their doctors before using this or any other drug.*

Omalizumab is another drug currently being used to treat seasonal allergic rhinitis. It is a manufactured antibody that works against IgE, which as previously discussed is an antibody specifically seen in the allergic response. Put simply, omalizumab decreases IgE in the blood, which is beneficial because the higher the amount of IgE in the blood, the worse the symptoms generally are. One of the problems for using omalizumab treatment for allergic rhinitis is that it must be given by injection; it is not available as an oral medication. This drug hasn't been widely discussed in the treatment of sinusitis, but IgE is closely related to the eosinophils that bind to the nasal membrane and which may be the primary culprit in chronic sinusitis.

Immunotherapy, also called desensitization or known as allergy shots, is sometimes used when medications and environmental changes do not provide relief for perennial allergies. It involves injecting doses, once or twice a week, of the relevant allergens, the goal being to eventually desensitize the person to the substances. The dosage amount gradually increases until a maintenance dose is reached, and the patient should show improvement within three to six months. Immunotherapy may last two to five years, and by the end, the patient should no longer have the allergies.

Medical literature shows that most experts agree that corticosteroid medications and antihistamines provide significant relief only about *half* the time. When surveyed, patients generally say they get poor or partial relief from the standard treatments. Given that dismal situation, trying one of the newer approaches is worthwhile.

LINKING ASTHMA, ALLERGIES, AND CHRONIC SINUSITIS-LIKE SYMPTOMS

I discussed asthma and allergies in relation to chronic sinus symptoms because these conditions so often occur in the same person, either by perception or in reality. In particular, allergies and sinusitis might be confused and treatment is thus unsuccessful, especially if antihistamines dry out the sinuses and further block the mucus flow. Of course, it is possible to have both conditions, and the symptoms may "bounce" back and forth, depending on the treatment used.

In looking at how a sinusitis-like symptom may evolve into a chronic condition or ongoing pseudo-sinusitis, it is useful to think of it as a cycle.

1. The initial event is an obstruction of the ostia, which means that normal movement of air and mucus in and out of the sinuses is blocked.
2. That means that a dam is blocking the "river of mucus."

Nasal inflammation that results from a viral URI, an allergic sinusitis, or both contributes to "reinforcing" or "shoring up" the dam.

3. Thickened secretions are unable to pass through narrowed ostia, and the secretions accumulate, thus beginning a cycle in which the stagnant pond develops, and new infections begin, or the onset of a new cold or an allergy attack causes unresolved infections to flare up.

TREATING AN INDIVIDUAL, OR TREATING A MODEL

Unless the cycle is broken, the possibility of chronic sinusitis is established—and it may be stubborn. For this reason, doctors may recommend treatment with anti-inflammatory medications, such as steroids or antihistamines. They are attempting to break the cycle, but really are treating a model, and this model fits the disease *as they define it.* In a sense, the symptoms have caused the creation of the model in the first place, but in some ways the list of symptoms is still in search of a disease. Unfortunately, there is no actual scientific basis for the model, but it provides a place from which to work to treat individuals.

Some factors are missing from the model. For example, chronic sinusitis is not the same disease as acute bacterial sinusitis, or even acute sinusitis-like symptoms. However, the jump from acute to chronic is often based on the number of infections or the length of symptoms; it has not been logically or clearly defined. For example, an infection may last for weeks or months, and several different antibiotics are tried. Or, a person might have four different infections over the course of a year, and each is cured. Are both situations chronic sinusitis? Is it sinusitis at all? Was the initial infection actually an infection? It is difficult to know for sure. On the one hand, chronic sinusitis is defined as "stubborn symptoms that won't go away," and on the other hand, it's defined as "having numerous infections."

The unfortunate consequence of having many infections or one seemingly unending cluster of symptoms is that efficacious treatment is not straightforward. No single study or protocol exists to confirm what will work in all cases. In fact, quite the opposite is true.

A NEW ANGLE ON CHRONIC SINUSITIS

The importance of fungi in sinus infections varies among medical literature. When tissue is removed during surgery it is sent to the lab and examined for irregular cells or bacteria. Based on lab results, a condition known as "allergic fungal sinusitis" (AFS) has been documented in a small percentage of cases, estimated at 4 to 5 percent. Many patients with chronic sinusitis, however, seemed to have fungal growths in the sinuses, unconfirmed by routine laboratory tests.

Keep in mind that, like the intestinal tract, the nasal passages have "good" bacteria and fungi that promote health. The nose is a warm, moist environment, which is what fungi need to flourish. However, since the lab testing yielded little concrete evidence about the role of fungi in chronic sinusitis, it was not extensively researched. For the most part, thinking about chronic sinusitis remained locked in the bacterial infection model. If we figured out how to get rid of the "invading" bacteria once and for all, perhaps chronic sinusitis could be managed and finally cured.

The newer thinking about sinusitis is that the problem may be found in the composition of the mucous membrane itself. Researchers at the Mayo Clinic in Rochester, Minnesota, discovered clusters of eosinophils (a type of white blood cell) near the surface of the membrane. Although our knowledge of eosinophils is by no means complete, it appears that they have granules of protein used in their primary role, which is to fight off invading parasites. This provided the clue that perhaps chronic sinusitis is not caused by a "foreign" substance entering the body, but may arise from an internal mechanism. This suggested that nasal fungi might be potentially important after all.

Most people have fungi in the nose, but in those with sinusitis, the fungi look misshapen. Researchers found that in sinusitis patients, eosinophils were clustered around the fungi. The involvement of both fungi and eosinophils is explained by looking at the function of the substances. Eosinophils release MBP (major basic protein), a protein that is toxic to parasites (such as a fungus), but MBP also damages the mucous membrane and cilia, potentially even destroying cilia. This secondary damage done to the membranes and cilia then allows bacteria to penetrate to the sinuses through the mucous membranes, thus causing these recurrent infections. It's as if the natural protections that block or destroy bacteria have been damaged by a mechanism in the body designed to deal with a different type of invader.

The fungi itself may be important, too. In 1999, the Mayo Clinic reported that fungi were found in the nasal mucus in 92 percent of patients with chronic sinusitis. A 2001 study demonstrated that patients with chronic sinusitis responded to the presence of nasal fungus with eosinophilic inflammation. On the other hand, in healthy individuals this immune response to fungi does not occur. This suggests that the key to solving the problem may be related to the immune system's response to the fungus. Therefore, treat the fungus, prevent the eosinophilic inflammatory response, and you may prevent this abnormal immune system response.

Questions still remain—there is speculation that the rapid and large increase in sinusitis and asthma might be related to antibiotics in our food supply, specifically that given to cows, pigs, and poultry. The theory is that these antibiotics may then cause the normal, healthy bacteria we need to be killed off, which in turn allows the fungi to grow. Remember that bacteria and fungi must be in balance in the body, and if we destroy the healthy bacteria along with the harmful, we open the way for overproduction of other microorganisms, even those the body needs in correct, balanced amounts. This doesn't come as any surprise to anyone given an antibiotic for a urinary tract infection, which is often followed by a secondary yeast (fungal) infection. This imbalance also can happen in the nose. This antibiotic–fungi connection is one reason that McDonald's recently moved to ban the use of meat from suppliers whose beef cattle are routinely given antibiotics.

Although the cause-and-effect relationship hasn't been thoroughly studied yet, a look at Amish communities is revealing. They grow food and raise livestock without antibiotics, and asthma and sinusitis is almost never seen among older Amish individuals who follow traditional ways. Conversely, these conditions occur more frequently among younger Amish people who have fallen away from traditional food production methods. Thus, it is possible that the long-term use of antibiotics in our food supply has a role in the cycle of symptoms.

In another study, fifty-one patients, all of whom had had multiple nasal surgeries, used antifungal nasal sprays, and thirty-eight reported feeling better and also used decongestants and steroid nasal sprays less frequently. This antifungal treatment should not be viewed as a fast cure, however. The idea is to reverse the adverse "environment" in the nose, restore balance, and gradually return to normal. Acute sinusitis infection would be treated with antibiotics, but the antifungal treatments would be used to prevent recurrence. This treatment also holds promise as a new way to view the disease and avoid the surgeries that so often seem inevitable. If you have been told that surgery is almost certainly in your future, consider investigating this newer information about the root cause of chronic sinusitis.

SUMMARY

1. Chronic sinusitis can be easily confused with allergies, so always investigate allergies as a cause of persistent sinusitis-like symptoms.
2. It is worthwhile to undergo allergy testing because identifying and controlling the allergy may resolve the sinus symptoms.
3. Use allergy medications only after consulting your doctor; antihistamines that may control allergy symptoms have a drying effect on mucous membranes and may leave you vulnerable to colds or bacterial infections.
4. Persistent sinus symptoms and repeated antibiotic use can make some people vulnerable to a type of fungal infection that may worsen sinus symptoms. Talk to your doctor about this new angle on sinusitis-like symptoms.

Chapter 6

Headaches and Sinusitis

Like the common cold and back pain, headaches are one of the "ordinary" human maladies; however, those who suffer from frequent, severe headaches are unlikely to think of them that way. The one good thing about headaches is there are successful treatments today that were unavailable decades ago. If we go back a few millennia, we can see that our ancestors weren't so lucky, and according to archaeological evidence, treatment for severe headaches appeared to include drilling a hole in the skull! Fortunately for us, most men and women who suffer headache pain can find effective treatments, once they determine what type of headache affects them.

It is sometimes difficult to determine the source of the headache pain, and it may be even more difficult to describe it. However, the location and the quality of the pain provide the clues to reaching a correct diagnosis and treatment. Headaches often are a symptom of other health problems, and these must be investigated, too.

The sinuses are located in some of the common areas affected by headache and facial pain. However, discomfort

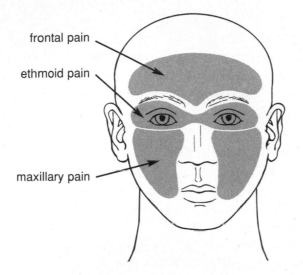

frontal pain

ethmoid pain

maxillary pain

Figure 6.1 Areas of sinus pain.

around the sinus regions may or may not indicate a problem with the sinuses. If we discuss the location and symptoms involved in any of the headache types, we can see parallels between sinusitis symptoms and certain types of headaches.

TYPES OF HEADACHES AND SITES OF PAIN

Classically, we believe the following about what are called sinus headaches or sinus-related pain (see figure 6.1).

- If the *frontal* sinuses are involved, the pain is experienced in the forehead.
- If the *ethmoid* sinuses are involved, the pain is experienced in the face and behind the eyes.

- If the deepest sinuses, the *sphenoid* sinuses, are involved (infections in the sphenoid sinuses are rare but serious), pain is experienced in the back of the head.
- If the *maxillary* sinuses, located in the middle third of the face, the pain is experienced in the area around the nose and eyes, as well as across the face. The upper teeth may be involved, too.

Remember that the maxillary sinuses are the most common site of sinus infections, and facial pain may be a symptom that an infection is present. However, the pain itself does not come from the fluid-filled sinus cavities, but rather, originates in the ostia and turbinates.

Sometimes headache sufferers say the pain feels like it is deep inside the head, as if it actually originated in the brain. However, the sources of the pain are the blood vessels, the muscles in the head, and the nerves surrounding the skull.

Of the headache types, sinus and tension headaches are the two most often self-diagnosed. This makes sense because if one has never had a migraine headache or had that concept introduced, all the nasal symptoms and eye tearing (lacrimation) appear to fit the symptoms of colds, sinusitis, and allergies. The term *sinus headache* is used incorrectly so often that the confusion about headache types is understandable. However, recent research shows that *98 percent* of those who believe their headaches were caused by sinus or allergy problems actually met the criteria for migraine headache developed by the International Headache Society (IHS). In addition, when given a short form of the Headache Impact Test (HIT-6), which measures headache disability, 84 percent of the individuals scored greater than 56, which means their headaches had substantial to very severe impact on their lives. Two-thirds of patients said they were dissatisfied with their current medical treatment.

Tension headache, like sinus pain with allergy, is one of the "advertised" human maladies for which there are dozens of OTC pain relievers. While it is true that taking an occasional headache medication should not cause concern, we have become too quick to medicate the so-called tension headache. This leads to overuse of pain-relieving medications. Unfortunately, this can lead to a "rebound" headache syndrome in which habitual use of pain medication interferes with the body's ability to deal with pain. Those who have nearly daily headaches may use OTC painkillers, thereby delaying any investigation into what is causing this frequency of headaches in the first place. Daily headaches of any kind are not normal, and I recommend seeing a doctor to determine why you have these regular and predictable pain episodes.

PAIN LOCATION HELPS DEFINE HEADACHE TYPES

With *tension* headaches (see figure 6.2), the pain *usually:*

- affects both sides of the head, but the location may vary;
- begins in the morning, and may begin during sleep, and worsen at night;
- may last for many days;
- has a steady ache, may worsen with manual pressure (such as rubbing the temples), and feels like a band on the head.

With *migraine* headaches (see figure 6.3), the pain *often* or *usually:*

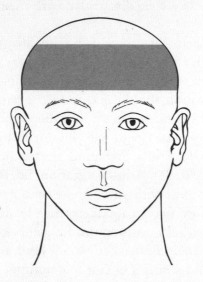

Figure 6.2 Tension headaches.

- occurs on one side of the head, is throbbing, and may feel as if it is penetrating the head;
- lasts hours or days;
- appears during "down" times, such as days off, vacations, and weekends;
- begins around menstruation in women of childbearing age;
- is accompanied by nausea, vomiting, flashing lights, phantosmia, or other sensory changes and sensitivities;
- is accompanied by flushing, sweating, runny nose, or congestion almost half the time.

With *cluster* headaches (see figure 6.4), the pain *often* or *usually:*

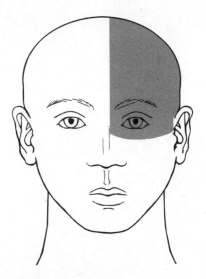

Figure 6.3 Migraine headaches.

- is located behind the eye, on one side, but may switch sides;
- feels piercing or burning;
- appears with no warning, with each "attack" lasting from thirty to forty-five minutes;
- leads to tearing, swelling, or drooping of the eye on the affected side;
- leads to nasal congestion on the affected side;
- leads to flushing and sweating on the face of the affected side;
- occurs seasonally and tends to start at the same time;
- comes in "clusters" of attacks over a day or for weeks, and then no attacks at all.

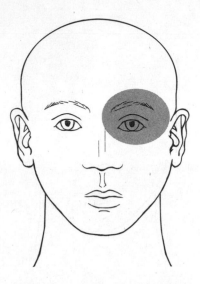

Figure 6.4 Cluster headaches.

With headaches that are traditionally believed to be due to the sinuses (see figure 6.5), the pain *often* or *usually:*

- is located above or below the eyes, may affect the cheeks and the area across the forehead, and may feel like pressure;
- is often said to be seasonal, but may occur at any time;
- is part of, or follows, an upper respiratory infection (e.g., colds or sinusitis), or occurs seasonally;
- begins in the morning and gets worse throughout the day;
- is accompanied by nasal congestion, discharge, postnasal drip, and sometimes fever;
- causes the areas of pain to be sensitive to the touch of the affected, painful areas;
- feels like pressure on the affected areas.

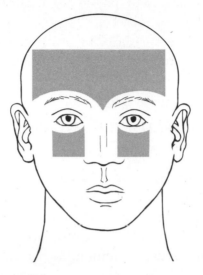

Figure 6.5 Sinus headaches.

The generally accepted *causes* of these four headache types break down as follows:

- *Tension headaches* are caused by poor posture, habitual jaw clenching and grinding the teeth, arthritis, emotional difficulties, depression, and external stressors (e.g., overwork and pressure and what many of us describe as having "a very bad day").
- *Migraine headaches* are caused by an imbalance of neurotransmitters in the brain, spasms or inflammation of the blood vessels in the head, stress, physiological reactions to certain foods, and—for women—changes in estrogen levels.
- *Cluster headaches* are caused by discharging of nerve fibers, by spasms, or from inflammation of the blood ves-

sels in the head and physiological reactions to certain foods, alcohol, or tobacco.

- *Sinus headaches* are caused by perceived pressure in the sinuses, nasal congestion caused by allergies, and blocked sinuses.

MORE ABOUT HEADACHES AND THEIR VARIOUS CAUSES

In terms of definition, headaches can be categorized as *primary* or *secondary*. Migraine, cluster, and tension headaches are considered primary because they are clinical conditions in and of themselves. Sinus headaches are considered secondary because they result from another condition, such as sinus infections or allergies. In addition, headaches occurring with other medical conditions such as a toothache, brain tumor, or head trauma are *secondary* headaches and do not fit into the predictable primary categories.

Those with severe headaches may initially be concerned about the possibility that they've developed a brain tumor. This is understandable because head pain tends to alarm most people. However, *headaches associated with brain tumors are relatively rare*. When headaches as a result of brain tumors do occur they're described as having a dull quality, rather than severe or sharp. These headaches can become worse with physical actions that raise fluid pressure within the brain, which include coughing, sneezing, and the strain that can accompany bowel movements. They often interfere with sleep and may be worse in the morning, and may produce serious neurological symptoms such as blurred vision, dizziness, or personality changes accompanied by lethargy and fainting episodes. CT scans and MRI are used to detect lesions or growths in the brain.

Headaches may also be an *early sign of hypertension*. These headaches tend to cause pain in the back of the head and may throb or pulse. Stooping, bending, or exercising may aggravate this type of headache because blood pressure tends to rise with these motions and with sustained exercise. Everyone should have their blood pressure checked regularly, regardless of the presence or absence of headache. If you do begin having headaches that match these characteristics, see your doctor immediately to have your blood pressure assessed.

Eye-related headaches produce pain just above the eye. This is another relatively rare cause of headache, and is sometimes thought of as eyestrain headaches. These headaches generally occur in the late afternoon after spending an entire day looking at the computer screen, for example, or following hours of doing other types of "close" work such as precision factory work or sewing. Pressure or pain in or around the eye should always be evaluated for the possibility of glaucoma or optic neuritis. The simple answer is that your vision may have changed and you need new glasses. On the other hand, halos around lights and eye pain may indicate acute glaucoma.

Facial pain and headaches can originate with dental problems. As previously discussed, pain in the upper teeth could be a sign of a problem in the maxillary sinuses. Temporomandibular joint dysfuction (TMJ) is another cause of headaches that may be confused with tension and sinus headaches because of facial and dental symptoms.

The temporomandibular joint "operates" the jaw, and problems arising in the joint can cause symptoms that mimic other conditions. Fullness in the ear, clicking or popping sounds in the joint, pain in the joint, facial pain, headache pain that cascades down the neck and shoulders, inability to fully open the jaw, tooth sensitivity and pain, and grinding the teeth at night (bruxism) all may be caused by TMJ. Misdiagnoses of TMJ dysfunction may include arthritis, tension headaches, ear infections, or sinusitis, because of the facial pain and ear pressure. But TMJ symptoms are associated with malocclusion, that is, a problem with the alignment of the teeth, either an underbite or an overbite.

One additional problem with TMJ is that a host of other conditions usually are investigated before considering dental-related causes for the symptoms. It is possible to have both sinus problems and TMJ syndrome, so I suggest seeing a dentist if your pain seems to fit the profiles for both tension and sinus headaches. Your dentist may refer you to a specialist who can suggest treatments. If flare-ups occur only occasionally and are mild, it may be enough to control symptoms with anti-inflammatory medication such as ibuprofen and aspirin. If symptoms are severe and frequent, then your dentist may recommend correcting the bite problem using specialized dental splints. Surgery is sometimes recommended but, unfortunately, often ends up unsuccessful because disease or abnormalities in the joint itself may not be the cause of the pain. Therefore, performing surgery on the joint does not correct the true cause of the pain, the bite abnormality.

Neuralgia is a term that describes a condition in which a nerve fires off abnormally, which then produces pain in that area. Neuralgia can occur anywhere in the body, but when it occurs in the face, it can be confused with pain of another origin. *Tic douloureux* (also known as *trigeminal neuralgia*) involves pain in the face and head.

As the prefix implies, the *tri*geminal nerve, which supplies sensation to the face, has three parts: one part serves the forehead, the second serves the middle face between the eyes and mouth, and the third serves the area below the lips. The pain from this condition is not the dull throb of certain types of headaches. It is characterized by its sharp, excruciating quality, and it tends to occur in sudden bursts (paroxysms) of pain that may last only a few seconds or minutes. This pain occurs most commonly in areas around the nose or cheek.

Tic douloureux patients tend to have a trigger zone, and the pain is triggered when the zone area is irritated. These triggers could include simple activities like shaving, chewing, or blowing the nose. Tests do not reveal damage to the nerve, so a diagnosis depends on symptoms and history. The condition tends to begin in midlife and become worse over the years, and some patients choose surgery to destroy the nerve pathway that causes the pain. Because the pain is severe, narcotic pain-relief medications may be required and sometimes antiseizure medication is prescribed. This condition is important in a discussion of sinusitis because the trigeminal nerve is the sensation pathway for the face, and pain perceived in the sinuses may be referred pain from other locations.

Headaches can occur with *pressure in the sinuses*. When air isn't replaced within the sinuses because the ostia are blocked, this creates a vacuum and results in negative pressure within the sinuses as compared with outside barometric pressure. Many things cause air pressure changes, for example, flying. Flying when you have a cold can make pressure in the sinuses even worse. Scuba diving may also cause sinus swelling.

Allergies may cause headaches, but many people assume they are associated with sinus headaches and are triggered by pollen, ragweed, and so forth. However, allergies or sensitivities to certain substances may induce a migraine headache. Fifteen to 20 percent of migraineurs have experienced this kind of headache trigger. It has been thought that these migraines occur only when exposed to certain scents, such as cigarette smoke or a particular perfume, because these substances act as allergens to susceptible individuals. However, it is just as likely that the substance is not an allergen but a direct chemical pain-producing agent.

Food allergies and their association with a headache tend to be less easy to spot, but you can try eliminating the foods such as wheat, dairy, eggs, nuts, shellfish, pork, and chocolate because these are the most common foods that trigger allergy headaches.

Headaches associated with environmental allergies can be treated with antihistamines, and if a stuffy nose accompanies the headache, a decongestant may be added. These drugs may also help relieve migraine pain. But remember that antihistamines are not helpful with sinus infections and colds and may worsen nasal symptoms because antihistamines dry the mucous membranes in the nose.

MIGRAINE AND SINUSITIS CONFUSION

In an article entitled "Headaches: With Special Reference to Those of Nasal Origin" (published in the *Illinois Medical Journal*), Robert Sonnenschein, M.D., writes, "One of the pitfalls into which many specialists stumble is to assign to the group of organs they are accustomed to treat any symptoms which the patient presents." He further discusses the problem of distinguishing sinusitis pain from pain from other causes and says, "The most definitive thing about the pains of sinusitis is the uncertain localization thereof. There is no characteristic localization of the pain or tenderness in involvement of any particular sinus." Finally, Dr. Sonnenschein concludes, "It behooves the rhinologist to remember that all headaches do not arise from intranasal conditions."

Dr. Sonnenschein's article might have been written today, but in fact the article in question was published in 1920! We still face some of the same challenges when we attempt to correctly identify the cause of a cluster of symptoms, of which headache is but one. One reason sinus headaches and migraines are confused with each other has to do with the anatomy and physiology of headaches.

With migraine headaches, the pain stimulates the nerve in the head that senses pain, the trigeminal nerve. (This is the same nerve that is irritated when you slice onions and then your eyes water.) This nerve passes into the base of the brain and stops at a structure called the nucleus of the trigeminal nerve. Here, the sensation is relayed to the thalamus, where the pain signal is processed. From the thalamus the pain signal progresses to the cortex (the surface of the brain), where the geographic localization of the pain, the intensity of the pain, and the type of pain (burning, stinging, sharp, and so forth) is registered and the sensation of pain is experienced.

However, *it is due to the firing of the nucleus of the trigeminal nerve that many classic sinus symptoms occur during migraine headache.* In response to the migraine pain, the trigeminal nucleus is activated and projects to the face and sinuses, causing the runny nose, nasal congestion, and watery eyes. Those with a history of migraine headaches may recognize these common symptoms of their headaches, but many other individuals might think they have a sinus headache and/or sinusitis. Three factors are important here:

1. A headache alone does not make the definitive diagnosis of acute or chronic sinusitis.

2. The one key symptom in the diagnosis of sinusitis is the presence of pus.
3. Clear discharge combined with headache pain is more likely to indicate allergies or migraine.

The path of pain explains why misdiagnoses are so common. An estimated *fourteen million* migraine sufferers go undiagnosed because they believe they have sinus headaches, due to the location of the pain and the sinus symptoms.

OTHER MIGRAINE FACTS

It's extremely important to learn about migraine headaches, because symptoms can so often be misdiagnosed. About 18 percent of women and 7 percent of men have migraine headaches. This means that about thirty million Americans have them, and about 20 percent have their first episode before age ten. Migraines last anywhere from four to seventy-two hours, so this is a potentially disabling condition. If we try to put a price tag on the condition, it easily runs into many billions of dollars annually, not only in direct costs of medical care and medications, but in lost work time and productivity. Those who have never experienced a migraine may have difficulty understanding that pain can literally be blinding and often leaves the sufferer alone in a dark room waiting for the medication to take effect. Migraine headaches are "notable" because of the disabling quality of the symptoms. History and other literature reveal that Julius Caesar, Thomas Jefferson, Sigmund Freud, Karl Marx, Lewis Carroll, Charles Darwin, and Edgar Allan Poe all suffered from migraine headaches. Before we had the term *migraine,* this kind of headache was sometimes called a "sick" headache, probably because of the disabling symptoms.

Migraines fall into two categories: *classic* and *common*. The classic migraine:

- usually comes on gradually;
- lasts from hours to days;
- is characterized by throbbing, one-sided pain;
- has a visual or sensory aura, which includes flashing lights, phantom smells, or other changes in smell and taste.

The common migraine:

- does not have an aura associated with it;
- is associated with loss of appetite, nausea, and sometimes vomiting.

Another type of migraine headache is the *hemiplegic* migraine, which is characterized by paralysis on one side of the body. In this headache the aura includes motor functions, which may continue even after the headache resolves. The *basilar* headache is a migraine that affects the base of the brain and produces symptoms that involve consciousness, such as confusion, loss of consciousness, mental stupor, or even coma. These two more rare migraine groups are not the type that are easily confused with sinus headaches.

SO MANY "SYSTEMS" CAN BE INVOLVED

Migraines are often referred to as vascular headaches because it was once believed that they are caused by constriction in the arteries in the upper part of the brain, possibly due to an increase of serotonin, one of the numerous neurotransmitters produced in the brain. The constriction was thought to be responsible for the visual changes, such as the flashing lights and moving, dark circular areas in the field of vision. Following the constriction, the belief was that the artery dilates because of the decrease in serotonin, and the action of the artery closing and opening caused the sensation of migraine pain. (It has since become known that blood vessel dilation has nothing to do with migraine pain.)

Two chemicals—tyramine and phenylethylamine—are found in many common foods, such as aged cheeses, chocolate, yogurt, buttermilk, and red wine. Nitrates and nitrites, used in curing processes, are found in foods such as hot dogs. The flavor enhancer MSG (monosodium glutamate) may trigger what has been called the "Chinese restaurant headache." However, this additive appears in many prepared foods, from hot dogs to canned soup. It may be listed as "hydrolyzed food starch, hydrolyzed plant protein, flavor enhancers, and natural flavors." Pay particular attention to all canned or packaged foods as well as seasoned salt products. Alcohol may act as a blood vessel dilating agent, which is why many individuals who suffer from migraines avoid all alcohol, not just red wine.

Some female migraineurs are vulnerable to the onset of a headache when estrogen levels fall just before the onset of menses.

Changes in atmospheric pressure may trigger a migraine headache in both males and females. The imbalance of body pressure and atmospheric pressure that occurs at about eight thousand feet appears to be the condition that initiates a migraine. Changes in temperature, humidity, barometric pressure, and rate of air flow and ionization may also bring about a migraine. In susceptible individuals, external sensory stimuli may act as a trigger as well. For example, many types of odors, certain sounds, and flickering or flashing bright lights may act as triggers. Many migraine sufferers are more vulnerable when they are tired or during or after physical exertion.

Years ago, many physicians believed in a psychological component to migraine headaches. In other words, they linked certain kinds of personality traits with migraine. More recent research, however, suggests no personality differences between migraineurs and non-migraineurs, although such psychological responses as irritability and anxiety may appear during the headache phase. This is not surprising, given the intensity of the pain experienced. Some also report lethargy and drowsiness after the pain subsides. Rarely, more serious psychiatric symptoms appear. Of course, like other headaches, stress is a component, so treatment should go beyond using medications to control pain once it begins.

After studying all the factors, it appears that migraine headaches can have hormonal, dietary, environmental, and stress components.

TREATING MIGRAINE HEADACHES

Effectively treating migraine headaches includes three important steps:

1. Prevention, which includes stress and dietary management.
2. Relaxation techniques and exercise, which are biofeedback mechanisms.
3. Use of medication. Unfortunately, drug therapies do not follow a one-size-fits-all formula. The challenge is to match the drug to the individual and the type of headache involved. The goal is to minimize drug therapy as much as possible while recognizing that it is

sometimes necessary to control the pain, or in other circumstances, prevent the onset of the headache. (Common medications used for migraine headaches are listed in the appendix.)

IF YOU ARE NOT SURE . . .

You may not be sure if you have sinus, tension, or migraine headaches, especially if you have a mix of symptoms. Furthermore, you may believe you have chronic sinusitis, and perhaps that is the diagnosis you have received and medical care and diagnostic procedures have focused on that problem. If treatment has not been successful, or if it involves more of the same, I suggest changing the focus and looking for a different cause of the symptoms. For example, it is possible that you have:

- migraine headaches that mimic sinus headaches, and may or may not include congestion and rhinitis;
- allergies and migraine headaches and the nasal symptoms lead you to believe you have sinus headaches and, therefore, sinusitis;
- asthma and migraine headaches. These two conditions often coexist;
- sinusitis symptoms *and* migraine headaches. The two conditions coexist in your case.

INVESTIGATING MIGRAINE AND OTHER HEADACHES

We already know that sinusitis is a diagnosis that may or may not apply, but once it is a label attached to you, your treatment follows protocols designed for that disease. However, since so many patients who believe they have sinusitis don't, there is a strong case for investigating migraine or tension headaches. Sometimes, shifting the focus can lead to a new direction.

Because of the overlapping symptoms of sinus and headache syndromes, you can begin doing the detective work by keeping a symptom diary, with an emphasis on headache and facial pain, along with other sinus symptoms. Your symptom/headache diary will answer the following questions:

- When did the headaches first begin?
- Where is the pain located?
- What are the location patterns, if any?
- How often do the headaches occur?
- How long do they last?
- What is the severity?

Do any of the following symptoms appear along with the pain?

- watery eyes
- nasal congestion
- runny nose
- dental pain
- mouth breathing
- olfactory impairment
- nausea or vomiting
- light headedness or dizziness
- fatigue or exhaustion
- muscle aches

Do any of the following make the symptoms worse?

- sounds
- lights

- smoke
- exercise, bending, or jarring movements
- intercourse
- straining with bowel movement
- coughing or sneezing

Do any of the following make the symptoms better?

- medication
- rest
- silence
- darkened room
- moving around

Simply answering these questions will help your physician evaluate your symptoms and match them with the most likely diagnosis. In addition, your answers will help you identify triggers to your headaches and perhaps other symptoms as well. Symptom diaries prove valuable for identifying allergies as well as looking for foods that trigger migraine headaches. For this reason, I recommend avoiding the obvious trigger foods (e.g., aged cheese, red wine, and chocolate), then recording all foods eaten over a four-week period. You may begin to see patterns that correlate the foods you eat with onset of symptoms. This information is valuable when you seek medical help to sort out your symptoms and receive the correct diagnosis.

The protocol used to evaluate headaches varies from physician to physician and among headache centers, but certain basic steps are essential. In addition to symptom and diet diaries and a complete medical history, a thorough headache workup will likely include such lab tests as:

- blood work, including lipid and iron levels
- thyroid function tests
- EKG
- urinalysis
- tonometry to rule out glaucoma
- CT scan or MRI (in some cases)

Questionnaires and other ways to measure pain and symptoms and rule out other disorders are used. These include:

- personality assessments (e.g., Minnesota Multiphasic Personality Inventory [MMPI])
- depression inventory
- a variety of headache-pain assessment tools

SUMMARY

Despite the overlap of symptoms between sinusitis and migraine or tension headaches, it is critical to remember that

1. Headache is not one of the primary symptoms of *chronic* sinusitis, and further, it has been suggested that chronic sinusitis does not *cause* headaches.
2. Treatments suggested for chronic sinusitis are bound to be unsuccessful if the true cause of symptoms, including the nasal symptoms, are caused by migraine or tension headaches.
3. If your symptoms are "stubborn" and fewer and fewer nonsurgical treatment options are suggested to you, I recommend looking into the possibility that you are experiencing undiagnosed tension or migraine headaches.

Chapter 7

Connecting the Loss of
Smell and Sinusitis

Sinusitis is frequently cited as a cause of smell loss, and when considering what I've called "true sinusitis," it probably is. However, sinusitis-like symptoms are probably not the cause of smell loss, and the situation can be quite confusing. Although the ability to smell is often overlooked, it is an important sense and one of our most crucial survival mechanisms. Equally significant, smell and taste make a fundamental contribution to our quality of life. These senses form part of the day-to-day sensory experience we often take for granted, especially when we sit down to an enjoyable meal. Our ability to taste depends on our sense of smell because about 90 percent of what we call taste is actually smell. *Olfaction* is the scientific term for the sense of the smell, and *gustation* is the term for our sense of taste.

I'm discussing the concept of olfaction and smell loss to raise consciousness about the sense of smell and changes that may occur with or without the presence of sinus disease. Far too often, people don't talk about their sense of smell even in this medical context. They may have a diminished sense of smell for all kinds of reasons, yet not mention it to the doctor at all. However, the sense of smell is intimately related to many quality-of-life and health issues and needs to be investigated far more extensively than it has been in the past.

As you already know, the nose is a complex and "busy" place, and includes odor receptors located at the top of the nose. Inhaled odor molecules travel to these receptors, triggering a complex process that allows us to recognize and respond to various smells.

An inability to smell has consequences for one's quality of life, regardless of the cause. Certainly, one of the reasons we have the sense of smell is to protect us from toxic fumes, smoke, and, for our ancestors, the proximity of potential predators and the detection of a potential source of dinner. In modern life we tend to think of our ability to smell as a kind of "bonus" pleasure in life. We literally love to sniff the roses and we'll inhale deeply when we walk past a bakery. In actuality, it's much more important than that.

Unfortunately, loss of the ability to smell has consequences for emotional well-being, which often has implications for those with chronic sinus symptoms. A strong link exists between psychiatric disorders and smell and taste disorders. For example, 96 percent of a group of forty-six consecutive patients meet the criteria for at least two psychiatric disorders. Among the most frequent was generalized anxiety disorder, dysthmia (a mood disorder), and obsessive-compulsive personality disorder. In essence, most of these individuals could be described as anxious and depressed.

We do not yet know why depression and loss of ability to smell are so often linked. It even offers a "chicken and egg" puzzle in that we can't say for sure which comes first. In my opinion, it is likely that diminished ability to smell most likely leads to the onset of depression. Depression could be a natural response to a loss of a bodily function, but the sense of smell isn't recognized as serious, so individuals aren't "cut much slack" when they complain about it. In addition, diminished olfactory ability is something that can creep up, and patients often don't realize what has happened for a period of time. It is also possible that the loss of ability to smell is a symptom of an underlying psychiatric disease. The answers to these questions remain unknown. If you have chronic sinus symptoms and can no longer smell, you may attribute your sense of loss and "feeling down" to the realization that you have a chronic illness. However, it may be that the inability to smell is contributing as well. Regardless of the cause, it has been demonstrated that loss of smell has a profound effect on quality of life, ranging from relationship problems, decreased sex drive, decreased social interactions, loss of olfactory-evoked nostalgic memories, and less enjoyment from social situations.

No one can say for sure why psychological issues such as anxiety tend to appear when smell loss has occurred. It may be possible that chemicals exist in the air that affect the brain and influence mood, not unlike a natural free-floating "Valium," for example. Theoretically, these chemicals influence us below the level of consciousness and when our ability to detect them is diminished, anxiety can result.

Although this is speculation, we do know that the sense of smell is our built-in danger detector. In an evolutionary sense, it detected the presence of dangers and of food sources before the other senses processed sensory signals. In modern life, the hazards might be fire and smoke, toxic chemicals, and gas

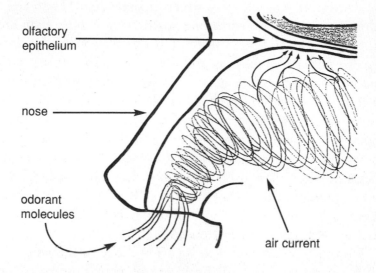

Figure 7.1 Breathing and the epithelia.

leaks. On an unconscious level, losing the sense of smell may lead to uneasiness; if the danger detector is no longer there to offer protection and a sense of security, uneasiness replaces it.

THE OLFACTORY SYSTEM

With each inhalation, odor molecules reach the *epithelia* in the olfactory "headquarters" at the top of the nose, just behind the bridge. Epithelia are mucus-coated membranes about the size of a dime. When you inhale deeply, air currents develop there that are best pictured as little tornadoes (see figure 7.1). When your nose feels stuffy, that means these nasal tornadoes are stronger than when your nasal passages are clear.

We have an *olfactory cycle*, which changes about every eight hours. Because of this cycle, one nostril is more open than the other at any given time. You can test this for yourself by closing one nostril and inhaling and then closing the other nostril and inhaling again. One nostril will feel a bit more stuffed up in comparison with the other. Your olfactory ability is better in the more congested nostril because the tiny tornadoes allow more odor molecules to be pushed to the olfactory epithelium to be "processed" and experienced as smells, pleasant or unpleasant, rather than just being carried deep into the lung. We notice the difference in the nostrils only when one is significantly more stuffed up than the other. Normally, this cycle goes on without your conscious awareness.

The olfactory or nasal cycle is part of the normal fluctuation in the shape and size of the inside of your nose based on swelling (or engorgement) and shrinking of the nasal lining. Lying on one side allows the nostril on top to open, which is reversed when you turn to the other side.

If you have a cold or a sinus infection or allergies, your nasal passages may become too congested and the odor molecules can't reach the top of the nose. Polyps can block odor molecules as well. When this happens, you may be unable to either smell or taste food, which is why food is described as tasting like cardboard.

Odor molecules caught in the air currents make their way to the olfactory membrane, which is about the size of the head of a pin and acts like a processing plant that sorts and classifies raw materials. It contains millions of olfactory receptors. Odor molecules then move through a thin mucous membrane where they bind to receptor sites on the olfactory nerve. We can tell one odor from another and identify the smells in our environment because odor molecules respond better at some receptor sites than at others. We have many millions of receptors and each links with odor molecules that match them.

When we breathe normally and easily, the airflow moves primarily along the middle and lower (inferior) turbinate. About 5 to 10 percent of the air is diverted upward in the direction of the olfactory cleft. If the mucosa changes in size it alters the air currents in the nose, which changes the little gales or tornadoes. This in turn influences the concentration of odor molecules in the nasal vault.

Research reveals that the sense of smell is better when we have some swelling and mucus secretion; olfactory acuity is worse when the mucous membrane is dry or shrunken. We can detect odors better when the membrane is slightly red, but when it is pale, the sense of smell is worse. In addition, odor molecules travel better in warm, moist air and a greater concentration of odor molecules reach the nose when moderate congestion is present. Nasal congestion is one of the many physiological responses we experience during sexual arousal. Assuming the existence of human pheromones, it is possible that the congestion allows a greater concentration of pheromones to reach the olfactory cleft. Presumably these pheromones enhance sexual arousal, which is part of nature's design to promote procreation.

The link between depression and smell loss is important. Breathing in odor molecules becomes an odor signal that ultimately reaches structures in the *limbic* part of the brain—our "emotional" center. The limbic brain is located below the *cortex*—our "logical" or cognitive center. The limbic lobe sits above the area of the brain stem that regulates unconscious functions such as breathing and digestion and other survival mechanisms we have no need to think about moment to moment. Our sense of smell is our most "feeling" sense because it is processed in the limbic center of the brain and is the only sense that provides a direct link to emotional responses.

An inhaled odor molecule has a direct influence on mood, and this link explains the powerful experience of nostalgic reverie, for example, or why some turn to comfort foods when they're ill. This connection also may contribute to swift and strong emotional judgments that can catch us off guard and leave us surprised by our own reactions. In other words, the brain may respond to an odor in the environment that we are not consciously aware of. Suddenly we find ourselves experiencing emotions that seem, at least for that moment, contrary to our "rational" self-concept.

Consciously and unconsciously, our sense of smell is part of our evaluation of people, places, and things. When we boil it down to our most basic evaluation, if something smells good, it is good. Likewise, if it smells bad, it is bad. When olfaction is impaired, as can occur with colds, sinusitis, and migraine headaches, and a host of other conditions, then such psychiatric symptoms as anxiety or depression may develop. Our sense of smell is so important because it plays a significant role in psychological well-being.

Even though much of olfaction remains a mystery, we do know it has an important role in shaping how we think, feel, and behave. For this reason, any impairment of this sense is bound to have consequences. Unfortunately, our sense of smell has yet to earn the respect afforded to sight, hearing, and touch, at least in the Western world, so its role in our health and well-being remains largely ignored. The adage "We don't know what we've got 'til it's gone" perfectly describes the general attitude toward this powerful sense. This is changing, however, as we continue to establish how powerful the sense of smell is, and how serious the consequences can be when it is impaired.

THE LANGUAGE OF SMELL AND TASTE

Smell and taste have their own language that helps describe the components and characteristics of each sense and the range of problems that can occur.

- The inability to smell is called *anosmia*.
- Reduced ability to smell is called *hyposmia*.
- An increased ability to smell is called *hyperosmia*.
- Perception of an odor that isn't present is called *phantosmia*.
- Distorted perception of an odor is called *dysosmia*.

Taste is similarly broken down into:

- *ageusia*, which is inability to taste;
- *hypogeusia*, reduced ability to taste;
- *hypergeusia*, increased ability to taste;
- *phantageusia*, a hallucinated taste;
- *dysgeusia*, distorted taste.

People who develop sinusitis-like symptoms frequently complain of reduced, distorted, or odd tastes. This is understandable when you realize that taste depends largely on smell. If you pinch your nose and pop a piece of chocolate in your mouth, you might as well be chomping on expensive cardboard. As previously stated, about 90 percent of taste is actually smell. In addition, taste is a misnomer in most cases. We're equipped to distinguish four categories of tastes: sweet, salty, sour, and bitter. We experience a variety of flavors through the retronasal mechanism. Odor molecules reach the olfactory bulb in two ways:

1. Odor molecules travel from the air to the nose, the orthonasal pathway.
2. Odor molecules travel along a pathway that starts at the back of the throat and moves up to the olfactory bulb, the retronasal pathway. (If you've ever laughed while you had liquid in your mouth and it came out your nose, you experienced this pathway in action.) When we chew food, odor molecules are released and move along the retronasal passageway.

What we describe as an odor is a combination of an odor molecule and a stimulus to the trigeminal nerve in the face. If you recall, this is the nerve that is stimulated when you slice onions. The nerve becomes irritated and triggers burning and tearing in your eyes; it is part of a protective mechanism that helps us sneeze and clear irritants and toxins before they harm us. Even if you can't detect the smell of an onion because your ability to smell is impaired, the trigeminal nerve detects an odor and responds. Think of it as a backup system designed to protect against various toxic substances. Smelling salts, which have a strong ammonia odor, provide another example of the way the trigeminal nerve is "irritated," thereby activating the part of the brain responsible for keeping us awake and alert. Tear gas also activates this mechanism. Exposure to smelling salts and tear gas results in burning eyes and difficulty breathing, a response that was initiated with an odor stimulating the olfactory nerve.

OLFACTORY INEQUALITY

Smell and taste acuity varies widely among individuals. Some people are born with a subnormal ability to smell, and they are "odor blind," the way some people are "color-blind." These individuals may not have any idea that they're missing something because no language talks about smell and taste in terms of a range. Subnormal ability to smell may run in families; I have talked with patients who discovered their "dull" olfactory acuity only when they moved into dormitories or had roommates who commented about smells. They were puzzled by the conversations because they didn't know these odors were present. *Congenital anosmia* is an inborn inability to smell and affects a small minority of the population.

A man may compare his sense of smell to his wife's ability to smell and assume that he has sinusitis or a nasal disease when really, by design, his sense of smell just isn't as acute. It is likely that women's superior olfactory ability is linked to the need to detect pheromones, especially during ovulation when a woman's sense of smell is at its best. This may seem insignificant today, but in an evolutionary sense it is probably part of the "reproductive imperative." In addition, female mammals can identify their young through odors, which is probably another evolutionary carryover that accounts for women's better olfactory acuity.

Although significant individual variation exists, we can say that olfactory acuity is better among women than men, and among the young versus the old. Just as other senses are affected by age, the sense of smell diminishes over time as well.

REASONS FOR OLFACTORY IMPAIRMENT

Olfactory dysfunction is a symptom of numerous conditions. Even in the presence of long-standing congestion and other nasal symptoms, do not assume that your sinus problems have caused your olfactory impairment. Other conditions linked with olfactory impairment include such things as:

- acute viral hepatitis
- hypothyroidism
- temporal lobe lesions (seizure disorders)
- Parkinson's disease
- Alzheimer's disease
- vitamin A deficiency
- head trauma

In addition, smell impairment is sometimes seen among patients who have had:

- coronary bypass surgery
- estrogen-receptor positive breast cancer

We also do not know the long-term effects of general anesthesia on the sense of smell, because the issue hasn't been thoroughly studied and it's unclear how long impaired ability to smell may persist after anesthesia is administered. In some cases, the symptoms can be reversed. For example, thyroid replacement treatment often reverses the distorted sense of smell and taste patients sometimes experience with hypothyroidism and other endocrine disorders. Inability to smell can develop for many reasons that have nothing to do with diseases of the respiratory system or sinuses.

Growing Older, Smelling Less

As I've said, olfactory acuity diminishes with age. Half of those over the age of sixty-five and 75 percent of those over age eighty have reduced ability to smell. There are many reasons this happens. As we age, we have decreased neurotransmitters (chemicals in the brain that regulate many functions), many of which are essential to olfaction. In addition, there is a cumulative effect over a lifetime of colds and respiratory illnesses. By age sixty-five the average person may have suffered hundreds of colds. In addition, incidents of minor head trauma may also have an effect over a lifetime. Smoking, even in the past, and heavy use of alcohol can also influence later olfactory ability.

In addition, some of the diseases that occur most commonly among the elderly, such as Alzheimer's disease, Parkinson's disease, diabetes, and hypothyroidism, affect the ability to smell. As individuals age, they are at increased risk for vitamin deficiencies because appetite tends to decrease and less food is consumed, and age also affects the ability to absorb nutrients from food. In addition, older people are likely to be on medications that affect smell. For example, antihistamines used for allergies and sinus conditions (and used sometimes incorrectly for colds and sinus congestion) may induce smell loss, even though theoretically they treat conditions (e.g., sinusitis) that affect smell.

Head Trauma or Injury

Although sinus disease is a significant cause of chemosensory impairment, most olfactory loss results from head trauma and the majority of that occurs in auto accidents. In these cases, the olfactory structures are damaged and the smell loss is often permanent—much of which could have been prevented by using a seat belt. The same is true for motorcycle and bicycle helmets. Without question, a significant portion of head trauma, with all its consequences, including olfactory impairment, could be prevented by consistent and universal use of seat belts and helmets.

Smell loss may also occur months after head trauma. Patients who were in an auto accident, seen in an emergency room, examined for head injury, and released begin to realize they can't smell or taste months later. For example, one of my patients had been assaulted and suffered multiple blows to the head, and it was six months before he realized he had lost the ability to smell and taste. In another case, a woman had been struck in the face and knocked unconscious on Michigan Avenue in Chicago. Nine months after the incident she noted the loss of smell and taste.

These serious events may have dire consequences. For example, the man who had been assaulted was a restaurant manager and because of his chemosensory losses was forced to find another profession. The woman who had been struck in the face was concerned about the inability to detect gas leaks, smoke, or spoiled food. In some cases, olfactory-impaired patients have sinusitis-like symptoms or a history of migraine headaches. They may also have experienced head trauma in the past. When the smell loss is investigated, however, the original head trauma isn't noted and the olfactory impairment is incorrectly attributed to sinus symptoms.

Sinusitis and Congestion

When air enters the nose, it descends into the lungs, but it's a journey that involves many twists and turns, and "road" conditions may change from moment to moment. For example, during a sinus infection or a cold, the olfactory epithelia can become inflamed and swell, which is how airflow to the olfactory bulb becomes blocked. The perception of smell depends on air reaching the olfactory bulb at the top of the nose. Sometimes reducing the blockage will improve the sense of smell, which is what usually happens after you recover from a cold. At other times, however, the composition of the mucosa—the thin lining—is changed and a barrier prevents the odor molecules from reaching "home," so even clearing and opening the nasal passages won't necessarily improve smell and taste.

About 10 percent of patients who believe they have lost their sense of smell may have normal olfaction when tested. When the problem is probed more deeply, these patients say that they experience not so much impaired as distorted smell. They may say that everything they smell is putrid or foul and they can't eat because their sense of taste isn't right either. A CT scan should be performed to investigate ethmoiditis, because even a single chronically infected cell can exude foul-smelling pus.

Sometimes people with chronic sinusitis complain about losing their sense of taste; however, tests may reveal their sense of taste is normal but their perception or interpretation of flavor is off. Likewise, some chronic sinusitis sufferers believe they have smell loss but when tested they are in the normal range. This could be a matter of episodic smell loss, or it could be a psychiatric issue. It is also possible that polyps are present, but the obstruction polyps cause is variable and results in only episodic smell loss. However, true sinus disease and structural abnormalities in the nose are common causes of olfactory loss. According to one study, this cause accounts for between 15 and 30 percent of individuals who are seen at a taste and smell clinic.

The secondary smell loss from nasal disease is called *conduc-*

tive loss, which means that the odor molecules cannot reach the olfactory cleft and the receptors. In this situation, the neural structure of the nose is intact. This condition, caused by inflammation or obstruction, can be easily treated, unlike neural damage resulting from trauma. Conductive damage can also result from the changes in the mucous membrane that covers the olfactory nerve.

It is possible that smell loss can result from sinusitis, even when no other symptoms are present. In other words, the one and only symptom of sinusitis may be olfactory impairment. The smell loss may come from inflammation or swelling in the ostiomeatal complex, but the patients may not experience nasal obstruction. Some patients may have had a viral infection or one or more episodes of what was diagnosed as a sinus infection, but subsequently experienced smell loss, even though the other sinus symptoms cleared up.

One reason sinus/olfactory symptoms are easy to confuse with each other is that the nasal vault at the top of the nose could be blocked, but the nose still functions normally and does its job of filtering, warming, and humidifying air; thus, the ability of air to pass through the airway appears normal. What this means is that patients may have lost their sense of smell because of a conductive problem or obstruction, but have no other nasal symptoms.

OLFACTION, MIGRAINES, PHANTOM ODORS

Some migraineurs report that their ability to smell undergoes a change at the beginning of a migraine headache. In some individuals an odor triggers the migraine. Olfactory hallucinations may also be part of the aura in migraines, and recent research reports that almost 11 percent of migraine sufferers report experiencing olfactory hallucinations. In addition, recent olfactory tests revealed that 18 percent either have subnormal ability to smell (hyposmic) or no ability to smell (anosmic). In general, olfactory dysfunction and migraines are both manifestations of irregularity in the limbic system. Sometimes the olfactory acuity changes during a migraine headache. For example, a patient with a cluster headache demonstrated hyperosmia, which is increased olfactory acuity, in the nostril on the same side as the headache pain.

Olfactory involvement in migraine headaches could occur for many reasons, including obstructed nasal passages and blocked airflow (often misperceived as sinus symptoms). Migraineurs with impaired ability to smell may be exposed to headache-inducing chemicals to an extent that the headache is produced, but the odor of the chemical isn't strong enough for these individuals to consciously detect it in the air. People with normal smell ability would avoid exposure to the odor and thus avoid the odor-induced headache.

On the other hand, odors may have potential to help ease headache pain. For example, the odor of green apple was studied for its ability to relieve headache pain, as well as for other conditions. Overall, green apple shows some ability to relieve headache pain, but only if the person finds the odor pleasing. In scientific terms, the efficacy of green apple as a treatment for migraine headaches was "hedonically dependent," or, simply put, "if you like it, it works."

Phantosmia (phantom smells) are generally unpleasant odors like garbage or mold. These can be precipitated by atmospheric changes, but they also can be resolved by changes in air pressure, such as diving into water, flying, or even standing on the head. These phantom odors can come and go, may be experienced in one nostril or the other, and may be eliminated by a change in air pressure. This could occur with sinusitis, but never assume that the smell is hallucinated because, as reported previously, a single chronically infected cell in the ethmoid sinuses can produce a foul odor.

Phantosmia often coexists with dysosmia, or distorted smell. This isn't common among those with conductive smell loss, but it is associated with postviral olfactory loss. In other words, a viral infection such as a cold can produce this distorted sense of smell.

Olfactory hallucinations can be extrinsic—coming from an external source, or it can be intrinsic, which means that the person believes that he or she is exuding the foul odor. This is known as *olfactory reference syndrome* and the perceived odor may come and go or be continuous. These individuals may withdraw from social life or they may change clothes more often than normal and maintain an intense concern about how they smell. This can be a self-isolating psychiatric disorder, and often becomes an identity: I smell bad, I must be bad.

This is the opposite of deliberately creating a bad odor in order to maintain distance, which is often seen among homeless individuals who use their own body odor to maintain their private world and keep others away. Their desire for isolation is often part of schizophrenia, a serious mental illness.

Bad breath—halitosis—which can be part of olfactory reference syndrome, that is, hallucinated, is a symptom of chronic sinusitis, so a concern about persistent bad breath should not be first viewed as a sign of a psychiatric abnormality when sinus symptoms are present.

TOXIC FUMES

A previously mentioned study conducted at the Smell & Taste Treatment and Research Foundation included 102 Chicago firefighters, and after adjusting the results for age and sex, almost half showed diminished ability to smell. Since it is generally believed that about 2 percent of the population has impaired ability to smell, this is a significant number. (The 2 percent figure is probably inaccurate; the actual percentage is probably higher.) A correlation also existed between the degree of impairment and the number of years on the job. Over 80 percent of the group said they wore protective masks while fighting fires, but olfactory acuity did not correlate with the use of the protective masks. Total number of years on the job was the key factor in determining the degree of loss.

Among those who had impaired ability to smell, 87 percent believed their sense of smell was normal, a typical finding for those who lose their sense of smell gradually. This is significant because the ability to detect odors is important for a firefighter, who most certainly needs to detect the odor added to natural gas. Gas leaks are a cause of fire, but are also a by-product of fire damage. Ironically, almost all of the study participants had gas furnaces in their own homes. Firefighters need their sense of smell to distinguish between odors such as burning wood and toxic chemicals, but fire departments don't test the ability to smell before hiring new firefighters. Because impaired ability to smell is linked with depression, reduced sex drive, and other quality-of-life concerns, the risk for firefighters increases as the years on the job accumulate.

This study found that 38 percent of the firefighters who showed olfactory impairment were the primary cooks in their households. Remember, most of these individuals believed their sense of smell was normal! (We once tested olfactory ability among chefs at 4-star restaurants and found that they, too, thought their sense of smell was normal, yet 30 to 40 percent showed subnormal ability to smell.) Among the firefighters, 34 percent of those with diminished ability to smell had experienced food poisoning one or more times—no surprise because testing showed that some of the smell-impaired firefighters could not distinguish between the odor of smoke and the odor of a dill pickle.

So, what does this mean? Certainly, it shows one more occupational hazard for firefighters, but it also gives us a look at potential consequences of neurotoxins or olfactotoxins (toxins affecting the structures that process odors and allow us to detect and identify odors). A wood fire produces as many as two hundred toxic chemicals, and many of these are known olfactotoxins. We can see that the potential for olfactory damage is great when we look at the combination of extreme heat, toxic substances, and physical exertion, which increases respiration. Smoldering wood, plastic, and fabric may still release fumes into the air after the "worst is over," thereby causing damage to olfactory neurons, especially because at this stage the firefighters may remove their protective masks.

Every year the United States reports two million fires, so the extent of toxic exposure to firefighters and others in the nearby environment may be greater than previously believed. This has consequences for olfactory ability, but also for sinus symptoms. Rather than jumping to the conclusion that sinus symptoms result from allergies or sinus infections, always consider exposure to toxic fumes.

Because firefighters are exposed to high levels of toxins, they could suffer from damage to the olfactory structures as well as experience irritation to the nasal passages. A single exposure to toxins could produce symptoms that mimic sinusitis, including migraine headaches. Congestion from colds, perhaps cigarette smoking, and a cyclical exposure to olfactotoxins could easily be misdiagnosed as sinusitis. Add headache or facial pain, which itself could be triggered by exposure to toxins, and you see a perfect example of how misdiagnoses could take place.

In other words, loss of smell could be due to chemical exposure, but it may be linked with sinus congestion, leading to a diagnosis of sinusitis. Given that diagnosis is based on symptoms, and antibiotics are given routinely, a firefighter might be treated for the wrong disease because the symptoms mimic other conditions. Sinusitis seems to cover all the bases, but the headaches or facial pain could be due to migraine, the smell loss could be caused by olfactotoxins, and the nasal congestion could be a response to toxic chemical exposure or caused by a migraine headache or a viral cold. Firefighters and anyone else who is exposed to toxic odors should have an accurate assessment of their sense of smell in order to take steps to protect themselves from damage by toxic fumes.

A host of toxins can cause smell loss: arsenic exposure, chlorine gas, trichloroethylene, lead, mercury, cadmium, and gold. Even a single exposure can damage smell and cause permanent loss. I saw a group of patients who had been exposed to a cloud of nitrogen tetroxide at one site and another group who had been exposed to chlorine gas elsewhere. Both groups suffered permanent smell loss. Exposure to chemicals can bring on the symptoms of sinusitis, nasal congestion, loss of smell, and headache.

DO YOU HAVE IMPAIRED SMELL OR SINUSITIS?

We cannot say for certain how many people with sinusitis have smell loss, just as it's difficult to determine the percentage of people with smell loss among those with any type of inflammatory condition of the nose. In a study of fifty-three individuals with conductive olfactory loss, 50 percent had rhinitis, sinusitis, nasal polyps, or postsurgical trauma. Those with intranasal polyps generally had greater smell loss. Almost half of those with conductive smell loss experienced fluctuation in ability to smell, sometimes based on activities that changed the level of congestion, such as exercise, exposure to steam, or using certain medications.

About 10 to 15 percent of the population suffers from allergic rhinitis. One study involving patients with active allergic rhinitis showed that 35 percent had measurable smell loss. Those in the study who had nasal polyps (usually the result of allergies) had worse smell function than those without the polyps. Looking at these numbers, it appears that many people with allergic rhinitis do *not* lose their sense of smell. In addition, the degree of disease does not determine the likelihood of losing olfactory acuity. The presence of polyps had a greater effect on olfaction. Smell loss can be a result of direct injury to the olfactory apparatus (e.g., the nerves in the epithelium). It is possible that scarring obstructs the nasal vault. It is unclear if the anosmia is a result of the obstruction or if the polyps have a direct effect on the olfactory membrane itself.

Patients with allergic rhinitis appear to have a degree of olfactory loss that is correlated with the presence of *eosinophilic cationic protein*, which is known to be a sensitive marker of allergies found in the mucus. The allergic response produces this protein and its presence is linked to some olfactory loss.

Strange as it may seem, olfactory testing is not routinely performed after surgery or as part of the diagnostic process for nasal and sinus disease and because of that, it is difficult to quantify the degree of smell loss and pinpoint the cause. Some patients complain of smell loss following rhinoplasty. One study that followed postoperative patients found that 10 percent had lost their sense of smell after surgery. The smell loss lasted for six to eighteen months, but all but one eventually recovered. These results were subjective, however, rather than based on testing. How individuals perceive their ability to smell may or may not be accurate.

In another study of one hundred patients undergoing surgery, researchers tested olfactory ability three to four weeks after surgery. Only eight had decrease in olfactory sensitivity, and one had no sense of smell. Another study showed that 3 percent had smell loss after an endoscopic procedure. In general, the risk of smell loss following surgery is considered to be just over 1 percent. However, nearly 10 percent of patients complain about the disruption of olfactory ability and, because testing isn't extensive in medical practice, it's hard to determine the actual risk.

Although sinus inflammation or infection, polyps, or rhinitis suggest the presence of conductive smell loss, simply looking in the nose with a nasal speculum may not reveal the cause. However, nasal endoscopy may detect disease in the vault or ostiomeatal complex that could otherwise be missed. In one study, almost half the patients who had conductive olfactory loss had normal findings on rhinoscopy, but nasal endoscopy showed pathology. This suggests that more extensive testing is necessary when investigating the source of smell loss, and endoscopic examination provides a better view of the sinus and turbinate structures.

In one study, twenty-four patients were tested for olfactory ability before and after surgery. Those whose sense of smell remained impaired after surgery were treated with topical steroid medication, and the twelve for whom the topical treatment didn't help were given oral steroid medication. Most reported improvement, but the side effects of the medication proved intolerable.

Studies have shown that among chronic sinusitis patients without polyps, 25 percent have olfactory loss; the percentage jumps to 83 percent when polyps are present. Among allergic rhinitis patients, approximately 15 percent report olfactory loss. Considering that 10 to 15 percent of the general population suffers from allergic rhinitis and about 14 percent of the population reports chronic sinusitis, millions experience smell loss. In addition, symptoms may come and go, particularly for those with allergies, and the loss may be gradual. It also may be worse among those who are allergic to numerous substances.

RESTORING YOUR SENSE OF SMELL

It is not known whether smell impairment occurs with sinus symptoms and disease because swelling in the olfactory cleft itself stops air from reaching the olfactory epithelium, or because inflammatory disease alters the chemistry of the mucus blanket. Typically, sinus disease leads to waxing and waning symptoms. In general, when patients take oral corticosteroids for sinus conditions, some note that their sense of smell returns, at least temporarily. Studies using topical steroids in the nose to reduce nasal swelling and restore the ability to smell have produced mixed results. In addition, oral steroid medication has side effects and in most cases, it is not recommended for continuous use except for particular diseases for which no other effective treatment is available.

Smell loss can occur after a viral infection, such as a common cold. Unfortunately, it is not known which nasal viruses cause damage that impairs smell even after the cold is gone. After most colds, the sense of smell returns to normal. Unfortunately, when it doesn't, steroid medication has not been shown to have an effect, and trials of vitamin A or zinc have not produced consistent results either. Postviral impairment usually occurs in older or middle-aged individuals.

If the sense of smell returns naturally after a cold or sinus infection, or with nasal steroids, antibiotics, antihistamines and/or immunotherapy (allergy shots), or endoscopic sinus surgery, then the ability to smell is intact. In other words, no permanent damage has been done to the nasal structures or nerves, as would be the case with some head and face injuries.

If you have a history of sinus symptoms and other possible causes have been investigated for your smell loss, then talk with your doctor about trying a course of steroid medication to see if olfactory ability returns. If it doesn't, a CT scan may help determine if the olfactory cleft is closed off or if an inflammatory problem exists that isn't causing other nasal symptoms. (MRI is not as good for identifying these problems because bony tissue is not as well defined.)

Steroid medication (also called corticosteroids) is sometimes used for patients with extensive nasal polyps and associated anosmia. One study reported that after a seven-day course of treatment, starting with 30 mg of prednisone and then tapered over seven days, patients reported improvement in ability to smell, and this correlated with the shrinking of the polyps.

However, the reports were subjective and no objective smell testing was performed.

A short course of high-dose corticosteroids improved smell loss in patients with non-allergic sinus disease. It is likely this worked because it reduced mucosal thickening or edema and allowed the odor molecule to reach the olfactory bulb. It also is possible that corticosteroids have a direct effect on the olfactory epithelium and have an anti-inflammatory effect. Olfactory function in one patient was maintained by low-dose oral corticosteroids; this became known as "steroid-dependent anosmia." But any treatment associated with long-term use of steroids is not recommended for most people.

Topical treatment with steroid nasal spray seems to have little adverse effect, so the topical application of corticosteroids to the nasal cavity is the first choice in treating olfactory dysfunction associated with sinus/nasal disease.

EVALUATING YOUR SENSE OF SMELL

Anyone with *any* of the symptoms for sinusitis, allergies, and migraine, or exposure to toxins, should be assessed for their ability to smell. As a patient, you must ask for this assessment and/or offer your own evaluation of your sense of smell because chemosensory testing is not routinely conducted as part of a physical examination.

If you are curious about the state of your olfactory ability, here is one easy test you can do. Have someone place in front of you two dishes of ice cream—one vanilla, one chocolate. Without looking at the dishes, have them hand you a spoonful of each. If you are unable to tell the difference between chocolate and vanilla ice cream without looking, you may have an olfactory deficit and should see your doctor to discuss the possible causes I've discussed in these pages.

SUMMARY

1. Though true sinusitis may contribute to or cause smell loss, sinusitis-like symptoms are most likely not responsible for chemosensory impairment.
2. The sense of smell is better when the nasal passages are moist and slightly congested; it is worse when nasal passages are dry and shrunken.
3. Olfactory impairment has numerous causes and is linked to many diseases.
4. Olfactory changes and impairment, including phantom or distorted tastes and smells, are part of both migraine headaches and sinus disease.
5. Exposure to toxic substances is a known cause of migraine headaches and may be a seldom-considered cause of sinus symptoms and smell loss.
6. Smell loss and some physical disorders are linked, which is why your sense of smell should be evaluated periodically. This is something you must monitor for yourself and ask for from your doctors because smell loss is not tested routinely.

Part II

PREVENTION
AND
TREATMENT

Chapter 8

―◉―

Contributors to Sinusitis

As we know, allergies can cause congestion, runny nose, and watery eyes. Allergies may be confused with sinusitis, and the same symptoms may appear at the onset of a migraine headache. That group of symptoms can be associated with a number of health concerns. However, congestion and other nasal symptoms can also be triggered by *neurotoxins*, and the symptoms are part of the body's protective mechanism.

For example, some people may believe they are allergic to chlorine because they have "allergy" symptoms after exposure to chlorine in a pool. I saw several patients who had been exposed to chlorine gas in an industrial accident in Las Vegas; they had developed sinus symptoms, among other exposure effects, including olfactory impairment, changes in the EEG (electroencephalogram), and changes in cognitive functioning. These were toxic effects, not a true allergic response.

Compare this with what we might call "swimming pool" or "water park" sinus congestion. The water in public pools and parks has such high chlorine content that many adults and children will develop colds and congestion after spending many hours in the water. When my children had colds immediately after spending the day at a water park I suspected that the chlorine had immobilized the cilia, which then slowed down the river of mucus and set up conditions for bacteria to grow. (Alternatively, they could have just been exposed to viruses from the other children there and developed acute viral infections.)

Similarly, some of my medical school classmates and I noted that we seemed to have colds and sinus symptoms during the semester in which we spent considerable time in the lab dissecting cadavers and inhaling formaldehyde. Like chlorine in a swimming pool, the formaldehyde immobilized the cilia. I also suspect that formaldehyde also reduces smell and taste, thus further mimicking sinus disease.

I once had a patient who had many allergies and frequently needed to go to the hospital for epinephrine shots for serious allergic responses. Then she suffered head trauma from a fall from a horse, which had left her with problems with smell and taste, along with some cognitive issues that included impaired thinking, writing, and speaking. When I saw her, which was about a year following the accident, all the symptoms had resolved, except for smell loss. At that point, she could be exposed to the same allergens that had caused serious reactions, including trips to the emergency room, but she no longer developed a response to them. This suggests that with certain substances, the conscious perception of the odor alone may be of sufficient magnitude to cause the allergic response. Thus, in some cases, allergies may be mediated through the sense of smell, meaning that the brain interprets the smell and then produces a secondary response—the allergy symptoms. Perhaps there is a lot more to allergies and what produces the symptoms than we have believed.

Certain odors such as cigarette smoke, paint, and perfume can trigger migraine headaches, and the sinus symptoms may be dominant in the episode. Or, the sinus symptoms may lead the person to believe he or she has an allergy to the substance, or that a sinusitis flare-up is beginning. In any case, the subsequent or concurrent headache is "interpreted" as a sinus headache or part of an allergy attack, when it could well be a migraine. This interpretation may well depend on the patient's previous diagnoses. For example, if you have been diagnosed with allergies or chronic sinusitis, then sinus symptoms are seen as part of that syndrome. But if your sinus symptoms were diagnosed as part of a headache syndrome, then the triggered symptoms will be viewed (and treated) based on what is viewed through that prism. This is why it is important to reevaluate the initial diagnosis if your condition is not improving.

Exposure to toxic fumes may be an underrecognized problem of sinus symptoms, headaches, and olfactory loss, among other symptoms. Firefighters represent an example of individuals who are regularly exposed to toxic fumes. Based on research at the Smell & Taste Treatment and Research Foundation, for this group of individuals smell loss is an occupational hazard that has gone largely unnoticed. We first saw six firefighters who were referred because they had complained about an inability to taste food; subsequently, we found that all six firefighters had lost their sense of smell, which was why their sense of taste was impaired. These six men provided a clue to a much larger occupational problem of chemosensory disorders caused by exposure to toxic chemicals.

MALODORS—OR BAD SMELLS AND FEELING BAD

Malodors—bad smells—can influence behavior, but they can also induce an allergic reaction and can contribute to accidents. Increased aggression was seen among school children who were exposed to bad smells coming from a landfill near their school. Teachers could document this because the children were exposed to the smell only when the wind blew from the direction of the landfill. Increased aggression was reported among inmates at a prison located near a garbage dump. Conversely, good smells seem to induce positive effects and make people happy. After two decades of studying the effects of smells on behavior, I sometimes wonder if the true aromatherapies are just the smells that make us happy.

The importance of malodors for sinus symptoms and headaches cannot be overlooked. Just as exposure to toxic fumes and materials can induce headaches and sinus symptoms, malodors should be considered a cause of these symptoms.

Malodors from such industrial sites as pulp mills may have direct effects on respiratory illness, such as asthma, or cause a permanent loss of smell. The increased aggression that occurs through exposure to malodors involves an adrenal response that raises blood pressure and increases risk of stroke or a cardiac event. Evidence exists that malodors can be linked to depression, insomnia, increased coughing, exacerbation of asthma, permanent olfactory impairment, and changes in immune system functioning. We tend to link pollution and sinus symptoms, but prolonged exposure to malodors is a serious issue, too (see chapter 7).

SUMMARY

1. If you think you have sinusitis and symptoms persist despite treatment, look for an environmental source of toxins.
2. Exposure to toxins can come from numerous sources, most commonly at home or work. Chemicals can enter your home in the water supply or they can be present in the air in your community.

Chapter 9

What You Can Do to Help Yourself

Chronic sinus symptoms, allergies, asthma, and frequent headaches are conditions that require ongoing, regular medical attention. If you have any of the conditions or recurring symptoms described in this book, you probably know what it's like to go to several different specialists looking for answers. Unfortunately, the need for regular medical attention may leave you with a sense of helplessness or dependency, which is why doing what you can for yourself can be empowering.

Ultimately, you are in charge of your health care. You gather the information and make the choices. By the same token, you are also in charge of your lifestyle, which, of course, includes steps you can take on a daily basis to stay well or improve your condition, which is the basic definition of self-care. Every day, you make choices about what you eat, how you cope with stress, and how you set up your home environment. You can enlist the help of your doctor or team of doctors. They can direct you to resources (books, products, or other clinicians) available to help you educate yourself about the lifestyle and self-care strategies that are right for you. Anyone with the symptoms and syndromes described in this book should be vigilant and proactive about self-care. In the end, it is a combination of self-care and medical care that will help you manage headache syndromes or sinus symptoms.

WATER—THE SIMPLEST THERAPY OF ALL

Most of us, even doctors, may groan when we hear again and again that we should be drinking at least six to eight glasses of water a day. For some reason, this seems difficult because we tend to consume so much coffee, tea, juice, and soda. Even though these are fluids, the body must still process—digest—these beverages much the way it digests food, so we need a steady supply of water. In addition, we tend to forget that our bodies are 60 to 70 percent water; we lose about a pint of water a day through exhalation and another pint through perspiration. We hear about the eight glasses as if it were a magic number, but in truth, water requirements are individual and based on weight. (See the formula that follows.)

As you know, water is essential for virtually every function of your body, and inadequate water intake can lead to numerous health problems, from faulty digestion and elimination to drying of the mucous membranes, which is our focus here. Those with sinus symptoms, including allergy and asthma, must stay well hydrated for the simple reason that the river of mucus depends on it. Water is absolutely necessary to keep the river flowing rapidly in order to prevent the formation of stagnant "ponds" in the sinuses, which as we've seen are breeding grounds for bacteria. In addition, to do their sweeping job efficiently, the cilia on the mucous membranes in the nose, sinuses, throat, and lungs must be kept moist. So, water is both a prevention strategy and a treatment. There is never a time when you can ignore your body's need for water.

It is also advisable to avoid iced drinks because cold temperatures may damage cilia and reduce the flow of mucus. So, avoid all cold drinks, including soft drinks or iced tea or coffee. Consume these beverages at room temperature or warmer.

To make the best use of water for prevention and treatment here are simple steps you can take:

Adequate Water Intake.   Use the following formula to calculate how much water you need per day:

Divide your weight in half and drink an ounce of water for every pound.

Example: A 128-pound woman needs 64 ounces of water, which is 8 glasses. If she exercises, she should drink more to replace what is lost through perspiration. As you can see, a 200-pound man will need considerably more water than a 128-pound woman.

Think moist!   Cold, wet compresses may reduce swelling in the sinuses because the cold will constrict blood vessels; therefore, use ice or cold packs to stop a sinus infection nosebleed. Moist heat may promote sinus drainage—the flow of the river mucus—and is soothing to the face and nose. You can use a hot water bottle (wrapped in a moist towel), or warm, moist towels alone, or a heating pad designed to create moist heat. These can be used on the face, especially over the forehead and under the eyes. You may prefer hydrocollator packs available in most drugstores. A warm shower also allows you to inhale steam, which helps thin the mucus and keep the mucous membranes moist. Two 10- to 15-minute sessions a day, one upon rising and one before retiring, may help reduce symptoms of congestion over time; this strategy may also be used as part of a self-care plan designed to prevent more flare-ups. Use these compresses as a home therapy for acute sinus infections as well.

Think hot and cold. This simple treatment may help reduce congestion. It calls for applying both cold and hot cloths to painful sinus areas on the face: two minutes of hot cloth application, one minute of cold cloth application, and then repeating the cycle three or four times, three times each day that you experience symptoms.

Think steam. Some individuals like to take regular trips to the steam room at their health club, and they don't wait for the first sign of a cold or nasal congestion. Steam helps keep the sinus passages open, so a session in the steam room is a valid prevention measure, and it is a treatment as well, because it can help thin mucus and open congested sinuses.

Some patients begin their day by adding moisture to the air in a very simple way. They put a pot of water on the stove and allow it to simmer. It's like delivering a quick shot of steam to the air and may help open nasal passages. (**Warning:** Some people lean over the stove and drape a towel over their head. Be careful with this method. First, be sure to turn off the stove before you lean over the steaming pot. Steam can burn the skin, but you'll also inhale gas fumes if the burner is on. In addition, there is a fire hazard involved with draping towels around your head and neck and then leaning close to an electric or gas burner. So be safe, turn the stove off and don't put your face too close to the rising steam.) Commercial steam inhalers are useful and are the high-tech, electric version of the simmering pot.

To scent or not to scent? Feel free to add grated fresh ginger or a stimulating oil such as peppermint, tangerine, or eucalyptus to the water. These are strong, stimulating scents. You can also add a teaspoon or so of Vicks VapoRub to the water. For many adults, the smell of Vicks is comforting because they associate it with childhood and being taken care of when they were ill. The olfactory-evoked nostalgic response is healthy and soothing.

Tiger Balm is an aromatic product found in drugstores and natural food markets and has a combination of "pungent" herbal extracts. A small amount can be rubbed on the temples or between the eyebrows. The stimulating smell can help clear the nose.

THE SINUS WASH

Sometimes called "nasal irrigation," this method of cleaning or clearing debris and bacteria from the nose, nasal passages, and sinuses can trace its roots back to ancient India, where it is part of an integrated system of care based on cleansing the body of substances that potentially interfere with health. For some, the saline sinus wash is much like simple body detoxification, similar to cleaning the teeth and gums, or eating a high-fiber diet and drinking plenty of water to promote optimal elimination. As a self-care strategy, it's relatively new in the United States, although I'm quite sure that individuals have probably brought this technique with them from many different cultures. It is both a prevention and treatment measure.

Even though saline nasal irrigation is easy, may be beneficial, and for the most part is harmless, I still recommend talking to your doctor before you run out to get yourself a nasal irrigator. First of all, rinsing the sinuses is *not a good idea when you have severe nasal congestion that blocks the nose*. Nor is it advisable when nasal polyps are an issue. I am always concerned about using any treatment or method that when misused could potentially harm the olfactory structures and affect the ability to smell.

That said, different methods of nasal washing may help relieve some kinds of sinus pain or nasal congestion, and your doctor can recommend the best way to use this self-care method if it is deemed safe for you. In addition, recommendations for the ratio of salt to water vary as well. Sinus irrigation is considered safe as long as you seek appropriate guidance about your individual situation and history. The goals of nasal irrigation are to:

- rinse away pollutants, allergens, and bacteria from the nose before they have the chance to settle in the mucus river or pond;
- promote thinning of the thick secretions that create stagnation in the river;
- wash away crusty secretions, pus, or bacteria;
- help prevent chest congestion caused by postnasal drip;
- help restore comfortable breathing by clearing congestion;
- moisten the sinuses and discourage or lessen inflammation.

The Low-Tech Way

A nasal irrigation device called a Neti pot (and similarly designed products) is low-tech, easy to use, and widely available in natural food markets and self-care and natural home-care catalogs and websites. It looks like a small, flat teapot with a spout. The exact ratio of salt to water will vary. However, in general, you're advised to use a quarter to a third of a teaspoon of salt (noniodized) dissolved in one cup of lukewarm water (bottled), along with no more than a pinch of baking soda.

You can also purchase saline solutions designed for nasal irrigation. These are called "isotonic" if they are formulated to mimic the same concentrations of salt in the body; they are called "hypertonic" if they contain a higher salt concentration. Hypertonic solutions are based on the theory that the increased salt content will relieve swelling in the sinuses by pulling fluid from the tissues. Hence, the swelling subsides and breathing becomes easier. However, this can also dry out already thin nasal membranes and perhaps damage cilia. Most OTC saline solutions follow the isotonic formula. In addition, avoid commercial saline solutions that have additives (e.g., antibacterial or antifungal substances and preservatives). The long-term effects of these additives are not known and they may interfere with olfaction and with other treatments recommended in your case.

The Neti pot, and the "look-alike" products, have a small spout that fits into the nostril. Simply rotate and tip your head over the sink and pour the solution into your nostril. The fluid rinses through your nasal cavity and after it drains through the other nostril, you spit out the fluid and repeat the process on the other side.

An ear syringe is another low-tech product. Turn it into a nasal syringe by filling the bulb with saline solution, then gently squeeze the fluid into each nostril. The solution will run out both sides of the nose and the mouth. A simple plastic squeeze bottle is also an inexpensive tool.

Your doctor may recommend using nasal irrigation once daily for prevention and two to four times a day at the first sign of a cold or sinus infection to help restore the health of the cilia following an infection.

Nasal Washing Goes High-Tech

One sinus irrigation product gives new life to your Water Pik, the pulsating device that uses water to massage the gums and remove loose food particles. Pulsatile Nasal Irrigator was developed by ENT specialist Murray Grossan, and it is based on the idea that pulsating irrigation is beneficial because the gentle rhythm and change in pressure achieved by the irrigation device may improve the sweeping motion of the cilia and improve blood flow to the sinus tissues.

The irrigator attachment is designed to fit the Water Pik and the "tank" portion of the device is filled with a saline solution (one formulated at home or purchased) and the *lowest pressure setting* is used to irrigate the nasal passages. One reason I recommend seeking your doctor's advice is that it is essential to use this device correctly, because blasting water into the sinuses with anything but very low pressure can damage the nasal and sinus structures, as well as the ears. Under high pressure, the saline solution could even exit through your tear ducts.

The future should see more research performed to assess the potential benefits of regular sinus irrigation. So far, this self-care method may be beneficial for those with congestion due to allergies and asthma, as well as for those with chronic sinus conditions. These devices may also help prevent colds and sinus infections.

Saline sprays.　Some OTC saline-only nasal sprays are available. These are nonaddictive and convenient because they are applied directly into the nose and can be used away from home. Do not use a spray solution that has any added substances, such as herbs or minerals, because their long-term effects on olfactory ability have not been adequately evaluated— in fact, many have not been evaluated at all.

Flutters and Strips

Give these nasal devices a try if your doctor believes they may help improve your breathing:

The flutter.   This device comprises a mouthpiece, a circular cone, and a stainless steel ball that sits inside the cone. The flutter is activated when you exhale into the mouthpiece, which activates the ball. The purpose is to create the "flutter," or oscillations, that in turn loosen mucus from the walls of the airways. This product is FDA approved for use by those with cystic fibrosis and bronchitis. You do not need a prescription to purchase it, but I strongly advise that you speak with your physician before considering it.

Nasal strips.   Nasal congestion and swollen sinuses often interfere with sleep, and the FDA has approved a product called Breathe Right that may help by gently opening the nasal passages. Simple in design, the strip fits over the bridge of the nose. A plastic strip springs back, which opens the nasal passage, allowing a greater degree of unobstructed airflow. These strips are available in varying sizes and can be purchased at any drugstore. They offer some usefulness for relief from snoring and also have been shown to improve the ability to smell.

CAN DIET HELP?

We now leap into confusing and treacherous waters, because we do not know nearly enough about individual responses to food, nor do we fully understand the role of each nutrient in building and maintaining health. If you have allergies, then you may have been tested for "trigger" foods, and if you have migraine headaches, you may also know which foods to avoid. However, for everyone else, it remains a matter of trial and error.

Choosing the right foods for you involves more than avoiding certain foods; rather, it requires a balance of basic nutrients designed to maintain health and prevent disease. As a start, I recommend avoiding overprocessed foods (because they include many additives), as well as sugar and alcohol, which both tend to aggravate fungal infections in the body. Those with migraine headaches and allergies may already avoid these and other foods (see chapter 5). If your doctor suspects that nasal fungi are involved in recurrent sinus infections, then eliminate both these substances from your diet.

What About Dairy?

Dairy has a bad reputation when it comes to sinus problems because dairy foods are said to be "mucus forming" or at least, dairy tends to thicken mucus, which is the opposite of the desired effect. However, researchers haven't demonstrated that dairy foods actually do thicken mucus, but subjectively, it is experienced as thicker. In other words, some people avoid dairy products at least during sinus flare-ups or colds because of their perception of thickened or increased mucus.

Addition, Not Subtraction

Rather than focusing on foods to stay away from, I prefer to talk about foods that help build your health, strengthen the immune system, and promote healing. For example, I recommend choosing *hot, spicy foods* because they tend to help keep mucus thin. This is much like what happens when you peel onions, which irritates the trigeminal nerve in the face, causing your nose to run and your eyes to tear. Temporarily, the mucus in your nose becomes thinner. In addition, different kinds of spicy foods are recommended for individuals with diminished ability to smell and taste.

- Cayenne pepper contains *capsaicin*, a substance that "irritates" or stimulates nerve fibers and seems to help clear nasal congestion.
- Garlic stimulates free-flowing mucus, and also contains a substance that is purported to be a natural blood thinner. Garlic is also believed to have antifungal and antibacterial properties and may help strengthen the immune system. Individuals with diminished ability to smell often add garlic to their food because it gives them some sensation of taste.
- Horseradish, like onions, may act like a natural decongestant.

In terms of day-to-day life, it might be worth trying spicy ethnic foods such as Cajun cooking, Indian dishes, and spicy Latin American and Asian foods—either in restaurants or when you cook at home. Experiment with these while you also avoid iced drinks, drink hot to warm liquids, and consume plenty of warm or room-temperature water.

Antioxidants

You have probably heard the terms *oxidation, free radicals,* and *antioxidant nutrients.* They are the subject of entire books and in the medical literature information is accumulating rapidly about the role of free radicals as "perpetrators" of disease and antioxidants as the heroes that come in and save the day.

Simply put, free radicals are molecules that have become unstable during the process of converting oxygen and nutrients to energy. In other words, free radicals are a by-product of the body's metabolic processes. Through oxidation, these molecules become like predators that try to normalize themselves by disrupting other molecules. Antioxidants act as scavengers who hunt for predators before they have a chance to harm the cells, and to that end, antioxidants are on twenty-four-hour search-and-destroy duty as they neutralize free radicals.

In recent years free radicals have been implicated in the development of many diseases, such as arthritis, cancer, heart disease, cataracts, and respiratory illnesses. Some of these diseases are linked with the aging process and might be called the degenerative conditions seen in advanced age. On a day-to-day basis, however, both the production of free radicals and their neutralization are part of an ongoing process in which our bodies are always engaged. Antioxidants are part of a protective army that tries to maintain immunity from bacteria and viruses and protects cells from damage.

In respiratory infections, free radical production has outrun its natural predators, or put another way, a weakness in the immune system has allowed bacteria or viruses to take hold and ultimately produce symptoms. When sinusitis becomes chronic, this signals an ongoing weakness, and one goal is to rid the body of the offending bacteria, which also means restoring the flow of the cleansing river of mucus, one of the body's natural weapons. A secondary goal is to restore the body's immune system's ability to maintain a protective shield. In a sense, this is a return to normalcy.

Our cells produce antioxidant enzymes, but the body also uses antioxidant nutrients from our food in order to prevent free radical damage. Every time you munch a carrot or eat an orange you are giving yourself a dose of antioxidant nutrients. An array of antioxidants occurs throughout our food supply, but we tend to notice the abundance of them in fruits and vegetables.

Vitamin C, vitamin A, beta-carotene (which the body converts to vitamin A), vitamin E, zinc, and selenium are all known antioxidant nutrients. In particular, vitamin A is of critical importance for maintaining mucous membranes in the respiratory system, from the nasal tissues to the lining in the lungs. As you know, the mucous membranes act like a shield that wards off invaders. Beta-carotene is one member of the carotenoid family; lutein and lycopene are two others. Without giving an exhaustive list, these important antioxidants can be seen by looking at nature's palette. In fact, the shades of green, yellow, orange, and red colors you see in the produce section at the supermarket are actually a display of antioxidants.

Bioflavonoids are a family of about four thousand compounds that provide the color in fruits, vegetables, and flowers. These bioflavonoids act as antioxidants, but they also work with vitamin C. In terms of respiratory disease and allergies, *quercetin*, a bioflavonoid, is important in reducing inflammation and helps prevent the cells from releasing histamine.

Many fruits and vegetables also contain vitamin C, which has natural antihistamine effects. It is one of the "supernutrients" for healing, which is why many people recommend taking it therapeutically in doses higher than the RDA (recommended daily allowances)—60 milligrams for adults. The RDAs for any nutrient represent a safe level of consumption as well as the minimal amount you need to protect you from certain diseases, such as scurvy in the case of vitamin C. In my opinion, taking many times that amount of vitamin C is safe for most people, so ask your doctor to recommend a supplemental dosage (usually from 500 mg to 2,000 mg) that allows you to reap the benefits of vitamin C without putting you at risk. The jury is still out on the benefits of mega-doses of this vitamin, but excessive amounts can cause stomach upset and diarrhea and may contribute to the formation of kidney stones. However, this is rare in the dosages under 2,000 mg.

Vitamin E is also a powerful antioxidant and specifically helps maintain the integrity of cell membranes. It may be one of the important nutrients in offsetting age-related changes. This vitamin also promotes production of T cells, whose function is to fight off disease. Vitamin E is found in many nuts and in fish such as salmon.

Vitamin E appears to work with selenium, a mineral that acts as an antioxidant to protect red blood cells. Selenium is naturally occurring in many grains and in seafood. Zinc, as previously mentioned, is one of the minerals that helps repair tissues and fights infection, but as previously cautioned: never use a nasal spray that contains zinc. Furthermore, newer studies have shown that oral zinc can impair immune system function, which leaves the user more susceptible to infections.

Good Fats

Essential fatty acids (EFAs) are necessary to maintain health, and they also work against inflammation through their role in producing a type of hormone called *prostaglandin*. We produce several kinds or families of prostaglandin that are involved in the inflammatory process in the body. The omega-3 fatty acids found primarily in fish oils and flaxseed oil, and the omega-6 fatty acids, gammalinolenic acid (GLA) and linolenic acid, are found in the oils of certain plants such as borage and evening primrose. These oils are available in supplement form, but you can also increase your intake of omega-3 oils by consuming oily fish such as salmon, mackerel, sardines, herring, and bluefish. You can also increase omega-3 fatty acids by adding ground flaxseeds to cereal or salads or using the oil in salad dressings.

A good diet is a critical part of self-care, so whether or not you currently take nutritional supplements, in my opinion you should:

- add an abundance of fruits and vegetables to your diet— a minimum of five servings. (A serving of most vegetables is about a half cup; a serving of fruit is usually one piece or one cup, or half a large grapefruit, for example.) Fruits and vegetables are nature's super-foods;
- educate yourself about nutrition and an optimal diet. Numerous books and nowadays, websites, exist that provide basic information;
- ask your doctor to recommend a dietician or nutritionist who can help you change your diet if need be and choose nutritional supplements. Don't make these choices on your own. Many people can benefit from dietary changes and supplemental vitamins and minerals, but you need a program that is right for you and does not put you at risk;
- try eating spicy foods that help thin mucus and relieve congestion.

Other Nutritional Strategies

A variety of enzymes are produced by the body and are necessary to break down and digest the foods we eat. Many different enzymes are sold over the counter as digestive aids. Two, papaya and bromelain, are sometimes recommended for sinusitis because they may help reduce inflammation. Papaya enzymes contain a high concentration of vitamin C. Talk to your doctor about papaya enzymes because proponents say they are useful as an additional treatment when you are taking antibiotics. Dissolving the enzyme tablets in your mouth, which is the way these are taken, may help shrink infected tonsils, allowing an antibiotic to better do its work. Papaya may also be useful in treating hoarseness and for reducing swelling in the eustachian tube. In all these applications, papaya works as an anti-inflammatory.

The bromelain enzyme helps digest proteins and inhibits the release of certain chemicals that cause inflammation. It also activates a chemical that breaks down fibrin, which is involved in the complex process of blood clotting. When fibrin breaks down, the tissues can drain and swelling is reduced. Bromelain can be purchased in tablet or capsule form, and it occurs naturally in pineapple.

What to Watch Out For

If you have allergies you may know to avoid certain substances that can cause an allergic response. For example, *sulfites* are used as preservatives in some foods and drugs. You may see different sulfite formulations on labels for commercial bakery products, salad dressing, pickles, sausage, dried fruit, beer, wine, packaged dried potatoes and other dehydrated vegetables, frozen and packaged shellfish, "chip" snack products, and some bottled corn syrup. These may be any one of the following: potassium metabisulfite, bisulfite, sodium sulfite, and sodium bisulfite. Sulfites may also be found on vegetables in salad bars. Look for these substances on food labels and on medication labels as well, especially if allergies are part of the sinusitis cycle for you. While you're reading labels, also look for food dyes, especially tartrazine—yellow food dye number 5. People with allergies and asthma should avoid this dye. Unfortunately, you will need to read many labels because this dye is found in many prepackaged sweets, such as cake, pudding, and frosting mixes, and in many other items, from cereals to packaged candy.

HERBAL REMEDIES

Just because a substance occurs in nature does not mean it is safe. This is certainly true for herbs and the herbal tinctures, capsules, and teas, which at one time were not easy to find. Now they appear in specialty food markets, drugstores, health food stories, and through mail-order catalogs and websites. Name an herb and you can find a source for it on the Internet. This is not to say that herbs have no potential value. In fact, herbal remedies were probably the earliest medicinal "product." They are still used throughout the world as primary treatments for various health problems and to promote well-being. But because they have not been tested in the United States using rigorous scientific methods and manufactured for consistent content, they will not be recommended in this book. For example, in one recent study, several "natural" OTC herbal products were found to contain a high lead content. In addition, just like drugs, they have side effects and are potentially harmful, depending on other factors. It's the "depending on" that is at the heart of the problem.

Some holistic physicians have taken an interest in herbal remedies and are knowledgeable about them, so if you are interested in using herbs, consult with one of them. When recommended by qualified physicians, herbal remedies may fall into a legitimate area of complementary therapies. However, do not take advice from self-trained lay practitioners or the Internet, because as you will see from even the brief descriptions that follow, *herbs that may be safe for some people are potentially harmful for others.* Some herbs are suggested as remedies for colds, flu, sinus conditions, allergies, and asthma, and others are recommended to strengthen immunity. Just as an example, the following are common herbs that are purported to be good for respiratory illnesses. You may see them marketed to treat various respiratory conditions.

Echinacea is said to enhance immunity and is marketed as an herb that helps prevent colds and flu. Although research results have been mixed at best, it is said to stimulate production of interferon and properdin, naturally occurring compounds that protect against infectious disease. Its effectiveness is time limited, so taking it continuously is never recommended. In addition, *individuals with autoimmune diseases should not use it.*

Goldenseal is often combined with echinacea and is said to be an anti-inflammatory that promotes the health of mucous membranes of the respiratory system. Two of its chemical compounds, berberine and hydrastine, are said to help fight sinus infections. It isn't recommended for people with blood sugar disorders.

Ginseng is available in many forms and is one of the "old" herbs used for a tonic and in treatment in various parts of the world. The trouble with it is that it is such a powerful herb that it causes all kinds of adverse reactions in certain people. It can cause headaches and rashes, increased blood pressure, asthma attacks, and heart palpitations. It may stimulate uterine bleeding or cause anxiety or insomnia. At one time it was thought that ginseng could improve memory (which would fit into the nearly universal and very old "folklore" that the plant has "restorative" properties, particularly among males, and promotes longevity). However, recent Scandinavian studies demonstrated that it was no more effective than placebo.

Two herbs may help relieve congestion and can be used in *cooking* to add spice:

Ginger has been used worldwide for many centuries. We know it as a spice, but it contains antiviral compounds, and is said to have antioxidant properties. It is also used as a digestive aid. However, I recommend using ginger as a spice only and not taken as a supplement. Ginger tea is widely available (and you can make your own with fresh ginger from the grocery store) and because it has a "bite," it is like spicy food and can help thin nasal mucus and keep passages open.

Garlic and garlic extracts have received attention in the last few years because garlic is purported to have antibacterial and antiviral properties. However, garlic (in undetermined amounts) acts as a *blood thinner*, which makes it potentially harmful to individuals on anticoagulant drugs. For this reason, do not take garlic supplements; however, ordinary use in cooking is not likely to pose a problem and may help relieve congestion and add flavor to food when your sense of taste is impaired.

Other herbs, including mullein, licorice, nettle, kava-kava, and myrrh, have been used for many centuries to treat respiratory illnesses. However, there are so many contraindications, from pregnancy to hypertension to fluid retention, that there is no way they can be recommended without knowledge of an individual's medical history and status.

YOUR ENVIRONMENT—KEEPING IT SIMPLE

I cannot "diagnose" the air quality in your home and pinpoint a particular problem, but there are simple steps you can take to set up an environment that helps avoid allergic reactions, asthma attacks, or sinus congestion. It's probably easier to think in terms of the broad categories, including:

- animal dander
- pollen
- dust/dust mites
- mold
- pollutants/toxic substances

To keep it simple, try to identify problem areas and take steps to eliminate them. Here are some ideas to explore.

If you have pets, keep them clean, do not have them sleep in your bedroom. Let non-allergic family members tend to the pets. Remember that even bird droppings and the feces of hamsters and cats are a source of mold and bacteria. For this reason, avoid litter boxes and cages. If you must be the person to tend to the pet, try to do so outside in open air.

If you smoke, stop! Talk with your doctor, because medications are available to help you and nicotine patches are sold OTC. Do not give up the quest to become a nonsmoker. If you don't smoke, but you live with a smoker, insist that smoking be an outdoor activity.

Avoid smoke of any kind, and that means fireplaces and outdoor bonfires.

Avoid exposure to pollen, which may mean staying indoors in an air-conditioned environment during allergy season—at least as much as possible. Keep the windows closed, change clothes after being outdoors, and consider installing an air filter.

Recognize that dust mites are everywhere, and they will invade your bedding, the carpeting, and so on. Dust mite waste is a major cause of allergic symptoms for millions of Americans.

You can try to minimize the problem, but it is not possible to completely eliminate it. You can wash your bedding frequently, use cotton or acrylic bed linen, remove carpeting from your bedroom, install specialized air filters to your air conditioning system that can minimize dust miles, as well as pollen and mold. Vacuum and dust often.

Mold loves damp environments, so use a dehumidifier in your basement to keep it dry, avoid mildew growth under sinks and in foundation cracks and the like, keep all your rooms aired and all surfaces dry, and do not hike or camp outdoors around damp vegetation. Avoid all outdoor areas where vegetation is decomposing. This is healthy for the natural world and is part of the life cycle of all living things, but mold spores are not good for you.

Avoid common products that may trigger respiratory symptoms—household cleaners, aerosol sprays, scented cleaning products and cosmetics, fumes from toxic substances, or common chemicals such as formaldehyde. The chlorine in swimming pools may trigger symptoms, too.

In addition to changing your household environment, pay attention to the levels of known pollutants such as ozone, nitrogen dioxide, carbon monoxide, and sulfur dioxide. Individuals with respiratory symptoms must be aware of the air quality in their communities and take steps to protect themselves as much as possible.

COMPLEMENTARY CARE

In recent decades, some physicians and patients have taken an interest in healing methods that complement conventional medical treatment. This trend goes by many names, including alternative and integrative care, but I prefer the term *comple-*

mentary because these methods are not part of what we understand as primary care today, but may complement conventional care. Unfortunately, few of these methods have demonstrated efficacy, although the anecdotal evidence is what raises interest in these modalities. Complementary care represents a contradiction of sorts. If the medical treatments available for chronic sinusitis worked well and led to a predictable outcome, then it would be unnecessary to explore these methods at all. But conventional methods have shown mixed results, and a few studies I've mentioned in previous chapters show that placebo works about as well as the active agents, or that "watchful waiting" was as or more effective than antibiotics for sinus infections. So, it is difficult to completely discourage experimentation with complementary therapies when conventional treatments show poor results.

Following are the most commonly sought complementary therapies.

Acupuncture

Acupuncture is one of the therapies in a health care system and philosophy that originated in China about three thousand years ago. In the United States, acupuncture, and all of Chinese medicine, is called "nontraditional," but it is the traditional health care system in China and other parts of Asia. To put it in the most simple terms, it is based on the idea that illness results from energy imbalance in the body; this life force energy is known as *chi*. The integrated system and philosophy is complex and involves the use of herbs, water, heat, and cold. Acupuncture is the component of Chinese medicine that has made its way to some conventional medical practices because it appears to have some value in controlling pain.

Acupuncture is based on the concept of stimulating energy points that exist along pathways, or meridians, in the body. This stimulation, traditionally using needles or heat, is intended to restore the natural flow of chi. (Acupuncture needles are extremely fine and insertion tends to hurt less than the familiar needle prick on the finger done for a blood sample. Traditionally, these needles were sterilized, but today in the United States, the needles tend to be used one time only and are then thrown away.) For reasons not well understood, acupuncture may increase production of endorphins, the body's natural painkilling chemicals. Its anesthetic value may correlate with the gate theory of pain, meaning that the acupuncture points along the meridians "close the gates" of the pathways that send pain messages to the brain.

A few studies have looked at acupuncture and allergies and sinus symptoms. One study looked at people with *allergic* rhinitis who received six acupuncture treatments. By the end of the sixth treatment, 50 percent reported that their symptoms had completely disappeared, 36 percent reported a moderate drop in symptoms, and 14 percent had no relief at all. Although the results were based primarily on subjective reports, blood studies did show a drop in eosinophils, which correlated with the degree of symptom relief or reduction. Recall that eosinophils are a type of white blood cell that mobilizes to fight invaders, and the Mayo clinic research found that they are elevated in the noses of those with chronic sinus symptoms.

Another study compared acupuncture and antihistamine treatments in forty-five patients with allergic rhinitis. Both methods brought some symptom relief, but acupuncture was slightly better and had a more prolonged effect. A study using acupuncture for thirteen patients with non-allergic rhinitis did not bring statistically significant improvement. More research is needed to sort out potential benefits of using acupuncture for a range of sinus-related symptoms. However, acupuncture shows some promise as a noninvasive treatment for allergic rhinitis.

Some physicians are incorporating acupuncture into their practices and I recommend seeking help from these physicians; as an alternative, ask your doctor for a referral to an acupuncturist with whom he or she is familiar and has confidence in. Do not go to a "storefront" clinic that offers acupuncture as one of many complementary therapies but does not have medically trained staff.

Acupressure Massage/Other Massage Techniques

The same points along the energy meridians can be stimulated manually, usually by applying pressure and holding it for as long as several minutes. This is an accessible way to try out the concept of acupuncture, and it is completely noninvasive and does not have any side effects. Some massage therapists incorporate acupressure into their massage methods; others learn *Shiatsu*, which is a type of massage based on acupressure and more important, on the idea of blocked energy as a cause of pain and illness. If you are interested in expanding self-care, you can learn to locate the energy points and apply acupressure on yourself. Other massage methods may use a variety of stroking techniques to induce muscle relaxation. They may very helpful, even if they are not focused on helping particular medical conditions or symptoms. It is possible that both acupressure and acupuncture may actually be helpful for muscle headache contraction or migraine headaches that are misdiagnosed as sinusitis.

Homeopathy

Samuel Hahnemann, a physician and chemist who practiced in the eighteenth century, developed homeopathy. The most well-known of Hahnemann's principles is the "Law of Similars," which is also known as "like cures like," or if a substance produces symptoms in a healthy person, then the substance will relieve symptoms in an ill person. The key to homeopathy, and the reason it keeps coming back into public consciousness, is the fact that the substance used to treat an illness is diluted so many times that no active trace of the substance can be detected in the remedy. For this reason, these remedies are considered safe. Consumers typically buy OTC homeopathic remedies for conditions that generally improve without any treatment, such as colds and flu symptoms. However, when scrutinized through scientific studies, these remedies are largely ineffective. Studies of homeopathic remedies used for treatment of migraine headaches and allergic rhinitis show that they perform no better than placebo.

Chiropractic

Chiropractic is based on the idea that disease is in large part the result of misalignment (subluxations) of the spine and treatment involves spinal manipulation. However, many chiropractic offices today offer nutrition counseling (and often sell nutritional products), massage therapy, and perhaps homeopathic remedies. (Osteopathy originally was based on a system of spinal manipulation meant to restore circulation. Osteopaths eventually moved into conventional medical treatment, including drugs and surgery, and are medical doctors. They should not be confused with chiropractors, who are not medical doctors.)

Treating diseases based on the concept of spinal abnormalities that appear on X rays is problematic for much the same reason that diagnosing sinus problems based on "mucosal thickening" is problematic. There appears to be no correlation between these abnormalities and symptoms. While chiropractic treatment can bring symptomatic relief for acute back pain, as a system of healing I find it lacking, especially for respiratory conditions and headache syndromes. If you are interested in nontraditional therapies, try exploring acupuncture and acupressure rather than pursuing chiropractic, because in my opinion those methods hold more promise for symptom relief.

Hypnotherapy

Hypnotherapy uses the mind to help heal the body, which is not a new idea. In fact, the powers of belief and suggestion are the doctor and patient's best friends, so to speak. My patients are not likely to improve if they have no faith in the treatment I recommend. Hypnotherapy is meant to engage the subconscious mind and "implant" suggestions that will aid healing. Sometimes it's employed to help overcome a habit such as cigarette smoking or to overcome a fear such as public speaking. Its effectiveness for those purposes is largely based on the subject's belief that it can be effective. Some research suggests that hypnotherapy is beneficial for pain relief, although its effects may be temporary, and it is dependent on the person's belief that it can help.

I view hypnotherapy as one of a group of relaxation/stress management techniques that many individuals find helpful. I do not believe one needs to suffer with a chronic illness to benefit from a system of induced relaxation. I recommend exploring meditation techniques, progressive relaxation, the "relaxation response," and self-hypnosis tapes. Literally hundreds of books, tape programs, and websites feature information about relaxation techniques, including self-hypnosis. Some find that the process of keeping a journal is a form of meditation.

STRESS—AGAIN

If you pick up any book on heart disease, hypertension, headaches, obesity, depression, insomnia, and a host of other conditions, you will read about stress. Even if you are hardy and healthy, you will be advised to educate yourself about coping with stress. You no doubt understand that stress is a key component in certain illnesses, and over a prolonged period of time, it can depress immunity.

Assuming that you experience chronic respiratory symptoms or headaches, which are stressful conditions, then you probably are painfully familiar with the ways stress can aggravate your situation. You have a condition that is stressful to your body and mind, and then stress can make the symptoms worse. Sometimes you're told to avoid stress—an impossible task. Your body is designed to cope with stress because life imposes stress on your body and mind. You might say all animal life is a complex matrix of chemical actions and reactions to external and internal stimuli. Trying to avoid stress is far too difficult, because that's like working against the natural order of things.

When you cope with symptoms that have developed into a chronic illness, like sinusitis, or you are subject to developing migraine headaches, or must avoid situations that trigger allergic responses or an asthma attack, then you have an extra challenge. You must adapt your lifestyle to allow for the adequate rest, exercise, and relaxation you need to stay well and symptom-free. There is no question that it can seem like a burden, and no one can tell you exactly what to do.

Some stress management suggestions have become almost a part of our cultural wisdom and life, and I offer them to you, not because they are new, but because they are reminders about what it takes to live a healthful lifestyle in a world filled with external and internal stressors. Consider the following, not as specific guidelines to help you cope with stress, but rather as topics to explore on your own or with your doctor. If you are trying to create a more healthful lifestyle, realize that you can't do it all at one time. Add stress management techniques one at a time.

Exercise

Next to choosing a healthful diet, exercise is the premier stress management tool and I "prescribe" exercise as part of the headache management program I designed for my patients. Countless studies have shown that adults who exercise live longer and better and its benefits for all major body "systems" cannot be overstated. It may seem impossible to exercise when you're congested, tired, and perhaps in pain as well. However, ask your doctor what exercise programs might be right for you, because the benefits for the circulatory system alone make it essential that you choose an activity you like and begin. Dancing, walking, and cycling help build cardiovascular health; yoga and Tai Chi promote flexibility, muscle strength, and concentration. Explore, find an exercise program that is safe for you, and just begin.

Meditation

I mentioned meditation earlier when discussing hypnotherapy, but it is worth repeating because it is an important stress management tool. Most people who meditate find it difficult to explain all the benefits they receive from giving themselves fifteen minutes to an hour a day to sit alone in a quiet space. Some meditation is focused and involves visualization or other mind-training techniques that relieve stress, promote relaxation, and improve sleep.

Schedules and Time Management

If you are overworked or overwhelmed, invest in a time management class or reevaluate your commitments. Individuals coping with chronic conditions must make choices and allow time for rest, exercise, and relaxation. This isn't an indulgence; it's a stress management tool that ultimately will improve your health. Almost every adult (and some children) I know have crammed schedules and always feel behind. No one can wrest you from the hold that overwork and overscheduling has on you. It's something you have to do for yourself. However, overwork is implicated in numerous health concerns, including respiratory syndromes.

Avoid Caffeine

Caffeine alone is a stressor because it is a stimulant that increases your blood pressure and heart rate, which are physiological responses to perceived danger and anxiety. Remove the caffeine and you remove a stimulus that elevates stress hormones in your body and keeps them elevated all day long. You will sleep better if you avoid caffeine.

Have a Massage, Enjoy Yourself

I previously discussed massage as a complementary therapy, but if you do not think of it as a treatment, then consider it an important stress management tool. If you enjoy massage but consider it an indulgence, reframe your attitude and list the ways it will help improve your health. Massage may be especially important if you suffer from insomnia, have a job that requires you to sit in front of a computer for many hours a day, or if you have difficulty relaxing.

Do whatever is necessary to create a lifestyle that promotes recovery and builds good health. If that means seeing a counselor to discuss some personal or family issues, then make the appointment now. Maybe it means taking a vacation or at least not overworking, or attending a time management or stress management seminar. Perhaps for you, stress and "lifestyle" management means joining a health club and consulting a fitness trainer who can help you design an exercise program. Maybe it means saying no to a request for your time. Most of us know what a healthful lifestyle is, but we don't focus on putting it into practice on a daily basis. Part of self-care is making a decision to shift your life and look in a different direction. Most people find that their symptoms improve when self-care and lifestyle issues become priorities. But these are decisions you have to make for yourself.

Chapter 10

When Surgery May Be Necessary

No one takes any type of surgery lightly, and although some sinus-related surgeries are often referred to as *minor* procedures, minor is a relative term. Yes, sinus surgeries are usually not performed under emergency conditions and the diseases for which they are performed are generally not life threatening. In addition, improved surgical techniques have dampened some of the fear of surgical complications and have reduced recovery time. But in the final analysis, minor surgery is usually not so minor to those for whom it's suggested. Every sinus-related surgical decision (except for those rare situations that qualify as emergencies) should be made based on the idea that surgery is a last resort, not to be taken lightly.

Endoscopy represents a major development in sinus surgery because it eliminated the need to cut through the roof of the mouth or along the bridge of the nose to gain access to the sinuses. The endoscope is a small telescope to which a video monitor is attached. The video display allows the surgeon to see a magnified picture of the sinuses. This surgical innovation gave rise to a greatly expanded field of sinus surgery because accuracy and safety provided greater rationale for working on the nasal structures in an attempt to correct structural abnormalities and chronic conditions. The ear/nose/throat specialists (ENTs) could be likened to a "corps of engineers" who work to keep the river of mucus flowing. Endoscopic procedures are designed to open the dams that may block the ostia or widen the channels through which the mucus flows. However, every time they remove tissue in the nose they are changing the nasal "terrain" permanently.

In many cases, sinus surgery is performed because medical treatment has not been successful and the sinus problems have become chronic. However, as discussed in chapter 4, chronic sinusitis remains a diagnosis in search of a disease. The definition of chronic sinusitis tends to be based on numbers of infections per year or the length of time an infection has persisted despite treatment. These arbitrary guidelines define the condition rather than defining it by objective anatomic abnormalities, specific pathologies, or well-delineated infectious origins. For example, strep throat is defined both by symptoms (redness and swelling in the throat) and an objective confirmation (throat culture). Sinusitis is a group of symptoms, but without objective measures to confirm it. This is why it is entirely possible that chronic sinusitis is not the true diagnosis in the first place. Therefore, the reasons surgery is being suggested may not be based on accurate assumptions.

You should consider the list of questions provided on page 174 to ask your doctor if surgery is offered as one option or is strongly recommended as a *permanent solution*, but first you should have at least a rudimentary understanding of the most common procedures and the reasons they are performed.

THE RANGE OF SURGICAL PROCEDURES

Surgery may be suggested for abnormalities of the nasal structures. One of the most common is the *septoplasty*, a procedure that corrects deviated septum, which is considered a cause of sinusitis. Deviation can be hereditary or the result of trauma to the nose, and when severe, it may cause a perpetually stuffy nose and sometimes snoring. The surgery widens the airway and removes or straightens the bent cartilage of the septum, which may have obstructed the flow of mucus and caused sinus-related symptoms.

Septoplasty is usually performed as an outpatient procedure and takes about ninety minutes. It is performed either under local anesthesia, or general anesthesia, in which case the patient is sedated. The "work" of the surgery takes place inside the nose, so no external incision is made and no bruising or swelling is visible. Following the procedure, the nose is packed to control any postsurgical bleeding. The packing is uncomfortable but not particularly painful and is removed in a day or two.

If rhinoplasty (cosmetic surgery to reshape the nose) is performed at the same time as septoplasty, there will be an external incision and visible bruising and swelling.

Deviated septum alone is not a reason to have this surgery, even if trauma to the face has caused the condition in adulthood. The surgery is performed only when the condition obstructs the nasal airways to the extent that you are susceptible to sinus infection and chronic congestion.

Rhinoplasty is a common surgery in our society and usually has few complications. However, another condition, nasal valve collapse, is seen among those who have had the surgery and also occurs among older people. The cartilage that supports the tip of the nose sometimes becomes weak and cannot support the air flowing into the nasal passage. To correct the problem, the surgeon takes cartilage from the septum or from the ear and adds it to the nasal tip. The procedure is called *nasal reconstruction*.

An older procedure called *Caldwell-Luc* directly creates an opening in the maxillary sinus cavity in order to strip away diseased tissue. The sinus is reached through a cut in the gum. It is still performed today and is usually an outpatient procedure. One reason this so frequently has a long-term failure rate is because a hole is made to drain the sinus, but not at the normal drainage site, the ostium; instead, it is made at another location more easily accessible for the surgeon. Thus, even after surgery, the cilia are still trying to push the mucus river toward the ostia. (The cilia don't know you've had surgery.) The ostium still remains occluded because it was never opened in the surgery. Even though the surgical trapdoor is opened, the river remains dammed up. (See figures 10.1 and 10.2.)

One of the most common reasons for surgery is to remove nasal polyps, the benign growths that often coexist with asthma and allergies. They become a problem because they have the potential to help create the blockages that slow down the river of mucus and lead to the stagnant ponds where bacteria breed. They can make the person feel chronically congested even in the absence of infection. In addition, nasal polyps are barriers to treatment such as the antifungal agents mentioned in chapter 4, so removing the polyps may enhance the effectiveness of some treatments.

ENTs also work on the turbinates using endoscopic techniques. As previously described, the turbinates in the nose can swell and obstruct the airways. Chronic infections, rhinitis, and allergies can cause the turbinates to enlarge, but then, the

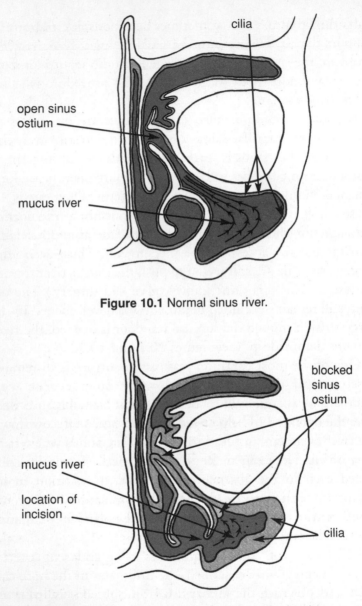

Figure 10.1 Normal sinus river.

Figure 10.2 Current still flows toward blocked ostium.

enlargement itself can create the conditions for bacteria to breed. Prolonged enlargement is called *turbinate hypertrophy* and outpatient surgeries to correct this condition are common. They include:

- *Partial turbinectomy:* The diseased areas are removed.
- *Submucus resection:* The bone under the turbinate is temporarily displaced and the turbinate is moved in order to open the airway.

Much of modern endoscopic surgery focuses on restoring proper drainage through the ostiomeatal complex (OMC) by removing diseased and thickened tissue that have created blockages.

SIGNIFICANT COMPLICATIONS

About 200,000 surgeries are performed each year in the United States using endoscopic techniques that were virtually unknown only a few decades ago. At one time, it looked like a breakthrough that would relieve the nasal symptoms of those whose lives had been severely affected by sinus infections and chronic congestion. Unfortunately, the results haven't been all that was hoped for. For many people, nasal surgery is not a onetime event. For example, partial turbinectomy may be repeated more than once, which means that less and less of the tissue remains intact. This can make the chronic symptoms worse. The turbinates humidify the nose and are part of the complex system that prevent infection by bacteria, viruses, and fungi. To remove turbinate tissue is removing one of the body's protective mechanisms. A Swedish ENT specialist called these "stripped" nasal passages the "empty nose syndrome" because so much tissue had been removed. In addition, it can take up to two years for the postoperative inflammation and damage to the cilia to resolve. Since nasal polyps tend to come back, the patient may not have completely healed from one surgery before another needs to be scheduled because of new polyps interfering with mucus flow.

When you consider surgery, realize that second surgeries are needed 20 to 50 percent of the time. One of the reasons the range is so great is that patients do not necessarily return to the same surgeon when their problems come back. In situations like this, it is difficult to define success. But you must understand that chances are about even that surgery is a temporary cure.

Other common complications include:

- *Impaired sense of smell:* Anytime a procedure involves entering the nose, you risk injuring the delicate olfactory structures. While it is true that sinus symptoms and polyps may impair the sense of smell, surgery may not correct the problem, and in some circumstances it can cause it or aggravate the sensory impairment.
- *Drying the mucous membranes:* When diseased tissue is removed, there may be fewer cells that produce mucus. This means less than the normal amount of mucus is produced and river of mucus turns into a mere stream.
- *Incomplete surgery:* This involves the risk of removing too little tissue rather than too much. This makes repeat surgery more likely.
- *Removing too much tissue:* In this situation, the nose is too open, which may cause excessive dryness, and in some cases, the patient has a burning sensation in the nasal passages.

Additional but rare complications with various nasal surgeries include damage to blood vessels and muscle tissue in the area around the eyes, potential to create a leak of cerebrospinal fluid, meningitis, and brain damage. Today's surgical techniques have reduced the potential for serious complications, but no surgery is completely without risk.

ASK THESE QUESTIONS *BEFORE* SURGERY

If surgery is offered as an option to treat your sinus symptoms, be sure to ask the following *general* questions:

Why this surgery, why now?

What other options are available?

What will happen if I don't have surgery?

What are the potential complications?

If you are told you have chronic sinusitis and your doctor means a chronic sinus infection, then ask about:

Treating the infection with a long course (several weeks to up to three months) of antibiotics given intravenously at home.

Using a topical antifungal spray either alone or in combination with the antibiotics.

Combining the course of antibiotics with a steroid nasal spray.

The possibility that the nasal symptoms are actually a sign of allergies, asthma, or are part of a migraine or tension headache syndrome.

If you are told you must have nasal polyps removed, ask the following:

> What benefits can I expect?
>
> Will the surgery improve my allergies, asthma, and congestion?
>
> Are the polyps likely to return?
>
> Are repeat surgeries common?
>
> Will my sense of smell improve or worsen?
>
> Can the polyps be treated without surgery?
>
> How long will the nasal inflammation last after surgery? (Be sure to raise the possibility that new polyp growth may begin before postoperative healing is complete.)

If you are told the surgery will involve removing diseased turbinates, ask the following:

> What benefits can I expect?
>
> Will the surgery improve allergies, asthma, and congestion?
>
> Are there permanent changes in the nasal terrain that may lead to problems in the future?
>
> Does this surgery sometimes fail to improve symptoms at all?
>
> Why does the surgery sometimes fail?
>
> Will normal mucus flow return?
>
> What postoperative self-care measures can help prevent the return of the sinus symptoms?
>
> Are the benefits long term or relatively short term, and

what percentage of patients require second, third, or even more surgeries? (In other words, what is the "worst-case scenario," based on studies within the field?)

In addition, always ask:

How many of these surgeries has the physician performed?

What percentage of *his or her* patients required additional surgeries?

What does the surgeon expect postoperatively (e.g., recovery time, not just from the surgical "injury" but the expected length of time before all swelling and inflammation is gone).

What other treatments or preventive measures does the surgeon suggest to prevent the need for surgery in the future? (In other words, what is the postoperative "game plan"?)

SUMMARIZING: ASSESSING YOUR OPTIONS

The purpose of asking so many questions is to uncover all your options and to receive a realistic assessment of the future course of the sinus symptoms if you agree to try surgery. Your questions involve:

- discovering a treatment option other than surgery
- uncovering another possible reason for your symptoms
- having a realistic understanding about the range of outcomes

- gaining confidence in both the procedure and the surgeon
- gaining an understanding of what the future could hold

Yes, sinus surgery may be your best option, but you will never feel certain about your decision unless you ask the relevant questions and examine the answers.

Chapter 11

When Children's Colds Become Complex

When we're born, we have only the ethmoid sinuses (located between the eyes and the cheek) and they are about the size of a pea. By age two, the sphenoid sinuses begin to develop and by age five they are large enough to appear on X rays. At about age four, the frontal sinuses begin to develop. Except for the frontal sinuses, which reach maximum growth by age twenty, all the paranasal (ethnoid, sphenoid, and maxillary) sinuses grow to their adult size by early adolescence. In practical terms, this means that it is not useful to use X rays to diagnose sinus disease in very young children.

ANOTHER COLD?

According to much of the medical literature, children typically have six to eight colds (also called upper respiratory tract infections, or URIs) each year. Although this number of colds is considered normal, about twenty-six million school days are missed each year because of colds. These colds are of varying degrees of severity. However, confusion exists about what constitutes a cold in a child. For example, no one knows how many times a normal child sneezes. Normal adults without a cold sneeze three times a day or less; anything over four sneezes could be a cold or could be an allergy. No such information exists that applies to children.

Children in day care centers or group day care in private homes are considered at slightly higher risk for contracting a cold. Teachers and day care workers often complain that they're more vulnerable to colds, too. Statistically, children experience the highest number of colds between ages three and six, and only a small number of childhood colds develop into sinus infections.

When you seek treatment for your child, remember that it makes no sense to treat recurring sinus infections if you don't address the possibility that your child has allergies, because the conditions may be closely linked. In addition, allergies may be a cause of confusion in "pseudo-sinusitis," or allergies may lead to true sinusitis. In colds and sinusitis, the nasal discharge is thick and yellow or greenish, whereas with allergies or sinusitis-like conditions, the discharge is thin and watery.

In adults, allergy symptoms include sneezing, watery eyes, and thin, watery nasal drainage. With allergies, it tends to be clear mucus, which distinguishes it from a sinus infection. Children with allergies also may have dark circles under their eyes, sometimes called "allergic shiners," and they may develop a habit of rubbing their noses in an upward motion (an "allergic salute").

Children with allergies often develop many symptoms that may or may not be confused with colds or sinus disease. For example, they may develop ear infections, chronic coughs, or asthma. Eczema, a skin disorder characterized by red, scaly patches, may be a sign that allergies are causing the respiratory symptoms.

If allergies remain untreated, over time mucosa in the nose and sinuses may swell, which causes a dam on the river of mucus at the ostia (the openings to the sinuses). This creates a stagnant environment that is a perfect breeding ground for bacteria and viruses. Thus, allergies can ultimately lead to colds and true sinusitis, but they may also mimic sinusitis and the common cold. Before children are treated for recurrent bacterial sinus infections and thus are labeled as having chronic sinusitis, they should be tested for allergies.

Allergies tend to run in families, so if both parents have allergies, a child has about a 65 to 75 percent chance of developing allergies, too. If you already know one child has allergies, then any suspicious symptoms that appear in another child should be quickly addressed because the odds are high that allergies are present. In addition, talk to your doctor about conditions that tend to appear with allergies, such as eczema or asthma.

Chapter 5 briefly described allergy tests (e.g., skin testing or RAST testing), which may be necessary to establish the specific allergies and the best treatment. They will also help differentiate your child's symptoms from sinusitis or frequent colds. In addition, the medications designed to control allergy symptoms may not be useful for children. An antihistamine that causes drowsiness in an adult may cause hyperactivity in some children. Nasal sprays that contain cortisone are not recommended for children under age six.

CAUSES OF SINUSITIS IN CHILDREN

Other conditions that can cause excessive nasal drainage in children include adenoiditis, or inflammation of the adenoids. The adenoids are located in the nasopharynx area. Children with enlarged adenoids may snore and speak with a nasal tone; however, they tend to outgrow these problems, because adenoids become normal adult sized by the late teens. The nasal tone usually disappears, along with the nasal drainage.

Infected adenoids may lead to a chronically runny nose. A sinus infection may be a secondary result. Likewise, enlarged or chronically infected tonsils can lead to sinus infections, too, because bacteria in mucus and pus can spread to nearby areas. Tonsils and adenoids are considered an "evolutionary remnant," that is, tissue that we can easily discard. However, in infants, the tonsils are important for development of T cells, which are a type of white blood cell that helps fight infection. At one time, tonsils were routinely removed in childhood because they were considered vulnerable to infection. Now tonsillectomies are uncommon, and tonsillitis is not a frequent diagnosis, proving that "fads" do exist in medical diagnosis and in surgical practice.

Exposure to secondhand smoke puts everyone at risk for respiratory symptoms, but some children, especially those with allergies, asthma, or any respiratory condition, are put at great risk for cilia damage and increased swelling and nasal irritation. If you are a parent who smokes, quit, and until you do, do your smoking outside your house and when your children are not around to be exposed to the smoke.

Small children are prone to putting objects (other than their fingers!) in their noses. Most pediatricians and ER doctors have dislodged a few buttons or peanuts or cotton balls from a child's nostril. The problem is, the object may not cause any problem when it's first stuck up the nose and the child forgets about it. A child may develop drainage in that nostril, and the foreign body in the nose can cause a foul odor. Therefore, if your small child develops drainage from only one nostril, then suspect that some small object may be lodged there.

Other possible, though less common causes include a condition called *choanal atresia* involves a blockage at the back of the nasal passages; a narrowing, rather than a blockage, is called *choanal stenosis*. This is diagnosed early in life because it means that the river of mucus can't flow backward through the nose and down the throat. Instead, the mucus pours out the nose and down the face. This problem is sometimes surgically corrected.

Facial abnormalities or cleft palate can interfere with normal sinus drainage. A rare condition called *ciliary dyskinesia* is characterized by abnormal movement of the cilia, and means that mucus drainage is slower than normal, setting the stage for the "stagnant pond" that may lead to sinus infections. If a child that does not respond to treatment for chronic infections or allergies it may be wise to look into this disorder.

You probably have heard of cystic fibrosis, a relatively rare but serious respiratory system disease that involves abnormally thickened mucus. It's a hereditary and debilitating illness that requires special care and usually results in early death. The risk of infection is always present because the thickened mucus blocks drainage.

Immunoglobulin deficiencies (immune system inadequacies) should be suspected in children who seem to develop many infections, regardless of location or type.

DIAGNOSING CHILDREN'S SINUS CONDITIONS

Diagnosing sinus disease in children can be difficult because the symptoms may have multiple causes, as is the case with adults. But to reiterate, the general signs and symptoms to watch for include the following:

- a cold lasting longer than seven to ten days
- constantly running nose, with thick green or yellow mucus
- postnasal drip, which then leads to a cough that is worse at night and interferes with sleep, or worse on waking in the morning. Children often are unaware of postnasal drip and they don't (or can't) talk about it. However, it may lead to a sore throat and bad breath (halitosis).
- The mucus stream can "overload" the digestive tract and lead to nausea and vomiting. Like adults, children can suffer from GERD (gastroesophageal reflux disease), a disorder in which the stomach acid travels upward through the esophagus, sometimes as far as the throat and nasopharynx. This can lead to a sore or hoarse throat. A child may not be able to talk about heartburn or a burning sensation in the throat, but if your child develops any of the chronic sinus disease symptoms, look into GERD as a possible cause. A hoarse voice, even in the absence of other symptoms, may indicate reflux disease.
- Children with sinus disease can be irritable or unusually tired. It's not unlike the "run-down" feeling adults describe when they have many colds or infections that linger and are resistant to treatment.

Fever is *not* necessarily a symptom associated with sinusitis, so do not use the presence or absence of a fever to draw conclusions about your child's condition.

Note: Watch your child for swelling around the eyes or any draining (of pus or nonwatery discharge) from the eyes. As with adults, this may be a sign of rare but serious complications of sinus disease.

In addition, your child should see a doctor if an ear infection, a severe sore throat, or a high fever develops; while we know colds can linger for longer than a week or ten days, even in children, be sure to watch these long-lasting colds for new or worsening symptoms. When it comes to children, it's better to err on the side of taking them to the doctor unnecessarily than risk complications from waiting too long.

TREATMENT

Naturally you want to help relieve your child's cold and sinus symptoms, but be careful about OTC medications and use these medications only if your family physician or pediatrician agrees they are useful. (A partial list is included in the appendix.) Consider the following factors:

- Oral decongestants may help relieve some nasal swelling and increase the airflow, but they may act on the brain and cause hyperactivity in some children.
- Do not use decongestant nasal drops for children under five, and if you give them to your older child, limit their use to no more than three or four days in order to avoid

the rebound effect, meaning that nasal swelling returns and the congestion cycle begins all over again.

- Antihistamines may be helpful if allergies are the issue, but their drying effect may thicken the mucus and prevent the river from flowing freely. Like decongestants they may cause hyperactivity or agitation in children rather than drowsiness.
- Analgesic medications such as acetaminophen (Tylenol) or ibuprofen (Advil) should be used only in children's doses, which are figured by both weight and age. Reye's syndrome is a rare, but serious complication associated with aspirin, so it is no longer recommended for children. (Analgesic medication of any kind may not be necessary to treat a cold or sinus symptoms.)
- Cough medications that contain *guaifenesin* will thin the mucus and make it easier to cough up.
- Read labels carefully and avoid combination medications, especially those containing antihistamines.
- A humidifier that provides cool air or a vaporizer that provides warm air may be useful to add moisture to the air. However, make sure your child cannot trip or fall and upset the vaporizer. Such an accident can cause scalding burns.
- Antibiotics likely will be considered for any cold that appears to have turned into a bacterial infection. They may be appropriate, but look for other causes of the symptoms before the congestion and infection cycle is considered "chronic," in which case your child may be given a longer course of antibiotics (three to six weeks). Ask you child's doctor about "watchful waiting."
- Sinus X rays are not performed routinely in children, and we want to avoid radiation exposure in any case. Besides,

in very young children, the sinuses are small and may not image well. If your doctor suggests any imaging tests, ask why he or she believes they will be of any help. What does the doctor expect to see? Will the findings have an impact on diagnosis? In certain circumstances, using MRI (magnetic resonance imaging) might be worthwhile and that technology avoids the radiation exposure involved in CT scans. However, even a routine cold can cause the MRI to be abnormal, so ask your doctor why he or she believes the MRI would be beneficial.

WHEN SURGERY *MAY* BE THE ANSWER

As a father, I know how difficult it is to think about children and surgery. It seems like such a drastic step, but severe complications of sinus disease call for aggressive surgical intervention; these complications include: orbital abscess (infection of the eye or the bones around the eye), severe brain infection, meningitis, or encephalitis. In these situations, the sinuses are drained as part of treatment—and it is an emergency!

Consider the surgical option if, over a period of time, your child's quality of life is compromised. Serious and "stubborn" nasal obstruction that aggravates existing respiratory disease, such as asthma or allergy, is a situation in which your child's overall health is adversely affected. Some research suggests that when nasal obstruction is removed, which "frees" the river of mucus to flow freely, children with asthma may use their inhalers less and have fewer trips to the ER.

Surgery usually is a last resort, and the anticipated benefits must justify the risk. The following are the procedures that could be considered:

- *Tonsillectomy and/or adenoidectomy (removal of tonsils and adenoids).* Enlarged tonsils and adenoids can be a "safe harbor" for bacteria. However, surgery to remove these tissues carries a risk. The problems are often outgrown, making surgery unnecessary.
- *Sinus drainage (antral lavage).* "Antral" is another name for the maxillary sinuses, and lavage means "to wash," so this procedure clears out infectious material and may also be used to culture the pus that is drained. Except in emergency situations, this procedure is rarely done.
- *Ethmoid sinus drainage (external ethmoidectomy).* This is done in emergency situations where sinusitis has affected the eye and vision and the ethmoid sinuses must be drained. These sinuses must be reached through the nose, so a small scar remains.
- *Correcting deviated septum (septoplasty/submucous resection).* Although these are outpatient procedures, they are rarely performed on children under age sixteen because while they may correct a defect in the septum, they may have an effect on the facial development.
- *Antral window.* This surgery involves creating a permanent opening or "window" between the maxillary sinuses and the nose. It is performed to correct blockage and help restore mucus flow, thus preventing the "stagnant pond" from developing during a cold. However, the new opening may close, so long-term success is not guaranteed. Furthermore, the cilia keep pushing the river of mucus in the direction they already know, which is toward the obstruction, so the window doesn't necessarily help very much. (See figures 10.1 and 10.2.)
- *Caldwell-Luc operation.* This procedure allows the sur-

geon to look directly at the maxillary sinuses. However, it involves making an incision under the gums. It is rarely called for and probably reserved only for severe cases of chronic sinus infection. It's considered risky because it may interfere with development of secondary teeth and with the growth of the maxillary sinuses.

- *Endoscopic sinus surgery.* This procedure is used to restore normal maxillary sinus function by removing diseased tissue and creating a "drainage" opening to the nose under the middle turbinate bone. Endoscopic surgery is used frequently in adults with chronic sinus symptoms and is considered a relatively safe surgical procedure. However, there is a risk of interfering with normal sinus growth or even damaging the developing sinuses, as well as causing loss of smell.

Any sinus surgery should be considered only as a last resort and after exhausting all other possibilities, unless a neurological or ophthalmological emergency exists. First, children almost always need a general anesthetic; this is always a risk, but especially for children whose brains are still developing. In addition, working on developing sinuses means risking permanent damage and creating scar tissue. If surgery is needed for any reason, ask detailed questions about postoperative care of nasal and sinus cavities and how frequently repeat surgeries are required.

Sinus symptoms can make a child's life miserable, so ask your doctor about all possible causes any risks involved with medications. If surgery is suggested, consent only in an emergency or after all other treatments have been tried and have failed.

Chapter 12

Frequently Asked Questions

I snore every night. I have nasal congestion, too. Do I probably have chronic sinusitis?

Snoring may indicate sinusitis, but the nasal congestion could be caused by asthma, allergies, or nasal obstruction associated with polyps or deviated septum. Snoring may be a symptom or warning sign of numerous conditions, including OSA (obstructive sleep apnea), which are periods in which breathing stops during sleep. Those with OSA may also have headaches, hypertension, depression, and daytime fatigue. Snoring may also be associated with conditions that appear unrelated such as heart disease, GI symptoms (heartburn), and morning headaches. Never assume that nasal symptoms are the cause of your snoring. Investigate the snoring phenomenon as a separate condition.

I've heard that if I take a decongestant for my headache and it gets better, that means my pain was probably caused by a sinus headache. Is this true?

This is generally not true. Decongestants and antihistamines are sometimes used to relieve migraine headache pain. It is likely that when congestion and pain go away after taking these medications the problem was migraine headache in the first place. Nasal symptoms associated with colds and sinusitis generally do not resolve with decongestants and antihistamines that are designed to relieve symptoms only. When the medication wears off, the symptoms return. However, these same medications usually relieve migraine pain and the pain does not return. In addition, sinus pain is a misnomer; pain we call a sinus headache is pain in the turbinates or ostia, or is really migraine.

I've been told I have Samter's syndrome, but that my sinusitis isn't part of that. What does that mean?

Samter's syndrome involves sensitivity to aspirin. It is a triad that includes asthma, nasal polyps, and aspirin intolerance. Aspirin is believed to cause nasal polyps in some people. Those with Samter's syndrome should never take aspirin, including any OTC decongestant medication combined with aspirin. Sinus symptoms may be associated with asthma and with polyps, but it is not part of Samter's syndrome.

I have a stubborn maxillary sinus infection. After three courses of antibiotics, my doctor suggested I have chronic sinusitis and should see a surgeon for possible endoscopic surgery. My dentist told me I have a tooth that requires a root canal and it could be causing the infection. Should I have the root canal before the surgery?

Infections or breaks in the upper teeth may cause inflammation in the sinuses that "behave" like a sinus infection. With your dentist fully informed about your history of sinusitis, I would try the root canal solution first. It *may* clear up your sinus symptoms, and even if you require surgery at a later date, any abnormality in a tooth should be addressed and the investment in the dental care may prevent more serious problems later.

What exactly is postnasal drip?

This frequently used term refers to thick phlegm that may feel "stuck" in the throat. It occurs because of reduced flow of mucus, causing it to thicken. During the night, many with nasal/sinus symptoms breathe through their mouth, causing the mucus "drip" to form a little stagnant pond in the back of the throat. This can irritate the throat and cause infection in the respiratory tract. The relief for postnasal drip is to restore the flow of the river.

I had nasal polyps removed two years ago, and now they are back. My sense of smell was virtually gone even before the first surgery. How likely is it that the second surgery will restore it?

Unfortunately, it is highly unlikely that your sense of smell will come back. If the first surgery removed the polyps that may have been blocking the olfactory epithelium but this didn't restore your sense of smell, then a second surgery has a low probability of success. However, I would talk with your doctor about investigating other reasons your sense of smell may be impaired. It is possible that sinus disease is not the cause. (See chapter 7 for a discussion of smell and causes of olfactory impairment.)

A friend of mine used to be a heavy cocaine user and now has chronic sinusitis and no sense of smell. Why does he have these symptoms five years after he stopped using the drug?

I once treated a young man who became caught up in a high-stress financial field and began using cocaine; this paralyzed the cilia in his nose and led to inflammation and a serious sinus infection that developed complications, including loss of vision caused by infection in the optic nerve. IV antibiotic treatment in the hospital cleared the infection and saved his sight, but like your friend, the damage to the nasal cilia was so great that the river of mucus is permanently "sluggish." Infections frequently recur and his sense of smell has never returned.

My doctor told me I have sinobronchial syndrome and chronic si-nusitis. What does that mean?

Although statistics are not exact, up to 70 percent of adults have coexisting lower respiratory disease such as asthma or bronchitis. The sinusitis may cause postnasal drip that irritates the throat and bronchi, which then leads to inflammatory conditions of the lung, such as asthma or bronchitis. Symptoms can be mild to severe, and the postnasal drip may cause coughing that interrupts sleep. The goal of treatment is to improve the sinus symptoms, thereby reducing irritation to throat and lungs that then triggers asthma attacks or coughing and wheezing. This situation illustrates how difficult it is to separate and isolate individual conditions that affect an entire physiological system.

My doctor told me not to bend my head backward when I use a nasal spray. She mentioned something called the Moffit's position?

The agents in nasal sprays reach the top of the nose when you lean forward, thereby applying the spray or drops to the nose in an upside down position (see figure12.1). If you've used nasal sprays in the past and they did not improve your symptoms, it is possible that the agent was ineffective because it never reached the top of the nose where the treatment was needed. If you are considering surgery, you might try these agents again, but this time using the Moffit's position. It is possible that this time treatment will be effective and you may be able to avoid surgery.

I enjoy scuba diving, but I have developed chronic sinus symptoms and asthma. Will continuing to dive make my symptoms worse?

Most likely your symptoms will continue to worsen because with changes in air pressure, vacuums are created within the sinuses. The vacuum causes the mucus lining to pull together, stimulating the nerve fibers that cause pain and setting up an internal

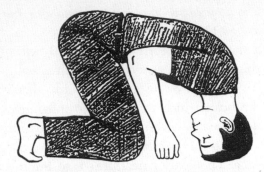

Figure 12.1 Moffit's position.

environment that is "friendly" for bacterial growth. What started as a vacuum can easily lead to another acute sinus infection.

I travel by air at least once a week, with the average flight lasting two to three hours. I have chronic nasal congestion and about two sinus infections a year that clear up with antibiotic treatment. What can I do before and during flights to prevent the congestion from becoming worse?

You can try taking a sedating type of decongestant before the flight, which will promote sleep as well as relieving nasal stuffiness. I also recommend chewing gum in order to keep the eustachian tube open, which allows pressure to be equalized between the air in the cabin and air in the sinus cavities. Drink plenty of water to keep the mucus river thin. Finally, avoid alcohol because it may lead to thickening of the mucus and act to paralyze the cilia.

Is there a way to determine if my immune system is impaired in some way, which is why I seem prone to frequent sinus infections?

If you have recurring symptoms, I recommend blood testing to measure certain immune system markers such as white blood cells (T and B cells and killer cells) and antibody levels. This testing may be easily missed in medical practice if patients undergo many different treatments with many different physicians. Several conditions, however, including mononucleosis and other viruses, such as HIV, can cause compromised immunity. The goal is to catch these conditions early when the problem can be corrected.

Pet dander bothers me, but my dog and cat are good companions and I've heard that pet owners are healthier and that animals help humans cope with stress. What should I do?

Reports in the popular press have discussed pets and stress management. I know that some organizations bring puppies and kittens to nursing homes for "pet therapy." A study at the Smell and Taste Treatment and Research Foundation was conducted to find out if pets had an effect on migraine headaches. Results revealed that having a dog or a cat did not reduce the severity, frequency, or duration of headaches. Yes, pets help make people happy, but unfortunately, allergies to pets can create problems in keeping the "river of mucus" flowing normally.

I have had chronic sinus symptoms for many years and I have seen numerous ENTs. Do you recommend seeing a neurologist to look at my symptoms from a different point of view? If so, will all the testing I have been through be useful or must I have all the diagnostic work repeated?

Yes, I would recommend consulting with a neurologist. Your previous blood and imaging tests will be very helpful in reaching a diagnosis, but a neurologist will want to do his or her own neurological history and examination. You may be asked to keep a symptom diary and your experience of your recent history will be viewed from a different angle.

Conclusion

———⊰◍⊱———

I hope that by now you have a greater understanding of the complex of potential conditions we may call sinusitis, but that perhaps should be referred to as a "sinusitis-like" syndrome. When all is said and done, true acute sinusitis is a relatively rare infection and if you think you have sinusitis you probably don't.

However, always keep in mind that *true* sinusitis is a serious condition and without question the medical literature supports beginning immediate and aggressive medical treatment. So, if you have *any* of the following symptoms, consider it a medical emergency and get to an emergency room. (This list of symptoms also applies to children.) You may require hospitalization with IV antibiotics.

- high, persistent fever
- swelling around the eyes, often unilateral, but swelling of both eyes is common as well. This swelling may make the eye appear to droop or bulge from the face, which are symptoms you must not ignore. (The swelling may or may not be painful.)

- tearing or discharge in the eye, along with a thick yellow or green nasal discharge
- neurological symptoms that *may* include such things as dizziness, visual or auditory changes, severe headache, and so forth. (Headache, facial pain, pain in the upper teeth may or may not be present.)

As I said, when these symptoms are linked to sinusitis they represent a medical emergency. When left untreated, the infection can progress and adversely affect eye structures and vision and spread to the brain or the optic nerve.

In the absence of these symptoms or true sinusitis, I suggest exploring the possibility that your group of symptoms is part of a sinusitis-like syndrome and you may benefit from exploring the following:

- *Asthma.* Half of those with asthma have symptoms associated with sinusitis.
- *Allergies.* Sinus-related symptoms are almost always part of an allergic response. In addition, asthma and allergies commonly coexist and individually or together can cause so many symptoms that they are labeled chronic sinusitis.
- *GERD.* As explained in this book, this common gastrointestinal disorder can cause sinusitis-like symptoms.
- *Migraine or other headache syndromes.* Migraine symptoms are often confused with sinusitis-like symptoms and may even be mislabeled as chronic sinusitis.

Talk with your doctor about these issues and open lines of communication in order to find the medical resources you need to reassess and treat your condition. In addition, I urge you to follow the commonsense self-care suggestions offered in this book. Your search for answers may take time, but your overall quality of life will improve if you make your health and well-being your priority.

I hope you find the solution you need to live fully with re-newed vitality.

Alan Hirsch, M.D.
Smell & Taste Treatment and Research Foundation
Chicago, IL

Appendix

Guide to Medications

"The desire to take medicine is perhaps the greatest feature which distinguishes man from animals."

So noted Sir William Osler, the famous Canadian-born physician who lived in the nineteenth and early twentieth century. Remember that taking medication for common complaints such as colds or temporary congestion is often unnecessary. Cold symptoms usually resolve on their own.

The following medications are listed by category, and in most cases, with active ingredients and brand names. The brand name list is not necessarily all-inclusive, but rather includes a sample of medications that are commonly used for colds, presumed bacterial sinus infections, allergies, and so forth. However, despite the astounding scope of existing advertising for these products, many are not useful or recommended for the millions of people with a variety of other medical conditions, including diabetes and hypertension. Therefore, I am not endorsing or recommending *any* of these medications for your individual symptoms. I recommend that you:

- ask your doctor if these medications are necessary and likely to either significantly relieve symptoms or hasten resolution of the problem;
- carefully read the labels for both common and less common side effects;
- read the label for optimal times to take the medication, since some may cause insomnia, while others may cause drowsiness.

OTC MEDICATIONS OFTEN USED FOR THE COMMON COLD AND SINUS INFECTIONS

- *Decongestants, oral.* These are taken to shrink nasal and sinus membranes, thereby reducing mucosal swelling and allowing easier breathing. Common oral decongestant products contain pseudoephedrine and phenylephrine, and possible common side effects of both substances include rapid heart rate, dizziness, insomnia, and nervousness, as well as a jittery feeling. Not recommended for nighttime use.

  If you are looking for a remedy to relieve cold and sinus symptoms, as opposed to allergy relief, be sure to avoid all decongestant products that contain antihistamines, because these dry the tissues and may make symptoms worse.
- *Sudafed and Triaminic.* These contain pseudoephedrine; they may also cause sweating, nausea, vomiting, and urinary retention.
- *Dimetane.* Contains phenylephrine (also used as an appetite suppressant) and may also cause headache.

Note: If you have diabetes, heart disease, hypertension, enlarged prostate, or thyroid disease talk with your doctor before taking any OTC product containing pseudoephedrine or phenyl-ephrine. Ask the pharmacist or your doctor about possible inter-actions with other drugs you are taking. Decongestant products for children are offered in syrup form, but do not use them with-out consulting a physician.

OTC DECONGESTANT NASAL SPRAYS OFTEN USED FOR COLDS AND SINUS INFECTIONS

- *Privene.* Contains naphazoline HCL.
- *Afrin.* Contains oxymetazoline HCL.
- *Otrivin.* Contains xylometazoline HCL.
- *Vicks.* Contains phenylephrine.

These sprays act quickly to begin nasal drainage, thereby providing fast relief. To avoid the rebound effect (*rhinitis medicamentosa*) discussed in chapter 2, use these sprays for no more than three to four days. If you decide to use these on a short-term basis, look for those with long-acting dosages (e.g., twelve hours).

The primary risk of these medications is the addiction to them that can occur if used more than three to four days. These may be useful for *temporary* use before and during air travel to prevent congestion.

OTC decongestants with expectorants may help keep mucus thin. These products add an expectorant to a decongestant. Expectorants help prevent thick nasal discharge that brings the "river of mucus" to a halt. They help loosen the phlegm in the bronchial tubes that can be cleared through a *productive* cough. The active expectorant ingredient is guaifenesin, as in:

Robitussin-PE Syrup

Triaminic Expectorant

Sudafed Non-Drying Liquid Caps

Because these include decongestants, the warnings for decongestant use listed above apply. These are available in both short- and long-acting varieties.

Cough suppressants have specific uses. Products containing dextromethorphan suppress the irritation and tickling that trigger coughing but do not suppress the beneficial, productive cough that clears the bronchial tubes. Dextromethorphan is found in NyQuil, Contac, and Robitussin. Possible side effects include dizziness, drowsiness, rash, nausea, and vomiting. Mental confusion and nervousness are rare reactions.

Cold medications may contain analgesics (pain relievers). Numerous OTC cold remedies are designed to provide "multi-symptom" relief. This means they add an analgesic such as aspirin, acetaminophen (the active ingredient in Tylenol), or an NSAID (non-steroidal anti-inflammatory drug) such as ibuprofen (the active ingredient in Advil and Motrin). Analgesic medications are meant to be taken for short-term problems, such as relieving temporary headache pain or the muscle and body aches that may accompany a cold. Each analgesic "family" has its own risks, and in general keep these warnings in mind:

- Aspirin may cause bleeding in the GI tract, and should not be given to children or adolescents because it is associated with Reye's syndrome (a rare but potentially life-threatening childhood condition).

- Acetaminophen may interact with alcohol and should not be used by those with liver or kidney conditions.
- NSAIDs may cause GI upset and bleeding.

If these analgesics are safe for you, a cold remedy containing a decongestant and an analgesic may be appropriate. However, be sure to read the labels carefully, because sometimes people unwittingly take aspirin or acetaminophen *in addition* to the cold remedy. They may also mix two different analgesics.

OTC decongestants with analgesics include Advil Cold and Sinus Tablets and Caplets; Alka-Seltzer Plus Cold and Sinus Medicine; Sudafed Cold and Sinus; Tylenol Sinus Tablets, Caplets, and Gelcaps; Sin-Aid Sinus Medication Caplets, Gelcaps, and Tablets; and Sinutab Sinus Medication.

Some decongestants include a cough suppressant and/or an expectorant. These products are recognizable because they are called "cough and cold" remedies or formulas. They act to relieve congestion, keep phlegm loose, and relieve throat irritation or a tickling cough. They may be marketed to relieve cold symptoms, flu, sinus symptoms, and coughs. They include such medications as Benylin Multisymptom; Comtrex Deep Chest Cold; Robitussin Maximum Strength Cough and Cold; Theraflu Maximum Strength Non-Drowsy Formula Caplets; Triaminic AM Cough and Decongestant Formula; Tylenol Cough Medication with Decongestant, Multisymptom; and Vicks DayQuil Liquid and Liquicaps.

Bear in mind that these are multisymptom medications and read the label for warnings that may make them inappropriate for you. In addition, the suggested dosage and length of usage varies, so follow the dosage directions carefully. Always check with your pediatrician or family physician before you give your child the pediatric formulation of these cold medications.

Cold and cough medications and decongestant nasal sprays may be useful to relieve symptoms of *acute* sinusitis. They are not recommended for any chronic condition.

Steroid nasal sprays are generally not recommended for colds and acute sinusitis symptoms. These prescription sprays may be useful for later treatment of sinus infections that required antibiotic treatment. Following the antibiotic treatment these sprays may help reduce swelling and hasten the healing of nasal tissues. They sometimes are used for chronic sinusitis and may help prevent osteomeatal swelling. They include: Flonase, Rhinocort, Nasonex, and Nasocort. Steroid nasal sprays do not have the side effects associated with *oral* steroid medications.

Saline sprays may be used prior to steroid sprays to prevent stinging or irritation. Steroid sprays may cause stinging in the nasal passages. Saline sprays can clear crusty nasal secretions and are used before the topical steroid medication is used. OTC saline sprays are available or make your own saline irrigation solution (see chapter 9).

ANTIHISTAMINES AND ALLERGIES

Antihistamines are useful for allergies, but may exacerbate colds and sinus infections. The problem may arise when the symptoms of a spring or late summer cold are misinterpreted as an allergic response and OTC allergy medications are taken because the symptoms appear to match. Antihistamines tend to dry the mucous membranes and slow down and dry up the mucus flow, so do not take them for colds and/or symptoms of sinus infections. Do not self-diagnose a seasonal or perennial allergy or self-medicate with OTC antihistamines.

If you have a diagnosed allergy and need occasional medication to relieve symptoms, OTC allergy medications may be beneficial. The OTC medications are often combined with decongestants, so do not take them if decongestants are not appropriate for you. These OTC products tend to cause drowsiness, so never drive or operate machinery or use tools at home when you take them. Common antihistamine products include:

- brompheniramine, Dimetane
- chlorpheniramine, Chlor-Trimeton
- clemastine, Tavist
- dephenhydramine, Benadryl

Combination decongestant and antihistamine products include Sudafed Cold & Allergy Tablets, Chlor-Trimeton 12 Hour Allergy/Decongestant Tablets (also available in four-hour dosage form), Drixoral Allergy/Sinus Extended-Release Tablets, Dimetapp Tablets, Contac Continuous Action Nasal Decongestant/Antihistamine, and Tylenol Allergy Sinus Caplets. Claritin (the OTC version of Clarinex) is also used for allergies.

Some effective antihistamines are available by prescription only. The three drugs listed below are generally considered nonsedating for most people. Prescription antihistamines include:

- loratadine, Clarinex (Claritin is the OTC version of this drug.)
- fexofenadine, Allegra (no OTC version available)
- cetirizine, Zyrtec (no OTC version available)

Side effects of Clarinex may include dry mouth, fatigue, and headache. Allegra may cause nausea, cold and flu symptoms, menstrual irregularities, and fatigue. Zyrtec may cause dry mouth and fatigue, and less frequently, sore throat and dizziness. Even though these drugs are said to be nonsedating, they may cause drowsiness in some individuals. Use them with caution.

Prescription corticosteroid nasal sprays may be useful for allergy patients; these include Beconase or Vancenase, Nasalide, Nasonex, Nasocort. These cortisone nasal sprays may cause bleeding or stinging (which is why the saline spray is recommended prior to use) and long-term use (more than six months) may cause fungal infection, or a perforation in the septum. These sprays should not be used during pregnancy.

The non-corticosteroid nasal spray cromolyn sodium (Nasalcrom) may be useful for allergy patients because it stabilizes mast cells. It is now available OTC. Nasalcrom is most effective if used prior to exposure to an allergen and may be started up to six weeks prior to the arrival of allergy season.

ANTIBIOTICS USED FOR SINUS INFECTIONS (PRESCRIPTION ONLY)

Chapters 3 and 4 discuss the efficacy of antibiotics for sinus infections. If they are prescribed, the antibiotics suggested for sinus infections include:

- Penicillin groups, which include the following generic names: amoxicillin, ampicillin, amoxicillin/clavulanate, dicloxacillin, penicillin;
- Sulfas and combination agents, which include generic names: sulfadiazine, sulfamethoxazole/trimethorprim (TMP-SMX), sulfisoxazole.

Side effects of antibiotics include GI symptoms such as nausea and diarrhea, possible yeast infections, and less frequently, skin rash and itching. Ask your doctor about taking acidophilus supplements while you're taking antibiotics. (Eating yogurt containing live cultures may help the GI symptoms as well.) These side effects do not mean you have an allergy to the antibiotic family. However, severe allergic reactions include anaphylactic shock. If you have a known allergy to one antibiotic do not take other antibiotics in the same family of drugs.

Less frequent reactions to antibiotics in the penicillin family include insomnia, muscle aches, sudden drop in blood pressure, hyperactivity, agitation, fatigue, tingling in the extremities, and other psychological and neurological symptoms.

Less frequent reactions to antibiotics in the sulfa drug family include sensitivity to light, loss of appetite, hives, dizziness, and confusion.

If your doctor recommends another family of antibiotics for a sinus infection, such as erythromycins (and macrolides), cephalosporins, tetracyclines, or quinolones, ask about the specific reason they are suggested. Based on reviews of treatment, the penicillin and sulfa groups appear to be most effective against sinus infections and these families of drugs are relatively inexpensive.

ORAL CORTISONE (CORTICOSTEROID) MEDICATIONS USED TO REDUCE INFLAMMATION (PRESCRIPTION ONLY)

These medications are used only when the potential benefits very likely outweigh the risks. The generic names for these drugs include prednisone, betamethasone, dexamethasone, and methylprednisolone. Prednisone is the most frequently prescribed of the oral steroid medications. The primary purpose is to reduce inflammatory effects. Taken for ten days or less, side effects are generally minimal. Dosages may sometimes be tapered from high to low, especially if used for longer than two weeks for chronic problems.

Side effects may include fluid retention and weight gain, bloating and facial swelling, GI symptoms (including ulcer), reduced immunity, hypertension, cataracts, increased bruising, and thinning of the bones (osteoporosis).

For obvious reasons, these side effects must be monitored carefully by your doctor. *Corticosteroid drugs may also interact with many different types of drugs, including antacids, diuretics, barbiturates, antiseizure medications (Dilantin), and oral medications for diabetes.*

DRUGS USED FOR MIGRAINE HEADACHES

Although this book does not deal primarily with migraine headaches, after reading the information presented here you may decide to seek further evaluation to determine whether your symptoms are related to a headache syndrome, particularly migraine headache. Therefore, familiarize yourself with the kinds of medications that could be suggested to you as part of a treatment plan for migraine headaches. The following is meant to be a *partial* list of common pharmaceutical approaches to migraine headache. However, treatment for migraine headache sometimes requires more than one medication and may include medications that both prevent headaches and treat those that occur. These medications have variable side effects, and experimentation often is necessary to find one that is well tolerated.

Some of the "first-line" medications used to stop the pain of migraine (referred to as "migraine abortive medications") are a class of drugs called *triptans*. They include sumitriptan, marketed as Imitrex, available as a nasal spray or an oral medication, and other similar oral medications such as Maxalt, Amerge, Axert, Relpax, Zomig, and Frova. The choice may depend on which is the best tolerated by the patient.

Narcotics (opioids) used to treat migraine include:

- Percocet (oxycodone and acetaminophen)
- Demerol (meperidine)
- Vicodin (hydrocodone and acetaminophen)

Falling into a class of drugs known as *anti-inflammatories*, naproxyn, marketed as Naprosyn, Naprelan, Anaprox, and Aleve (available OTC) may relieve headache pain. Taken daily, these medications may help *prevent* daily headaches; they may be suggested to prevent menstrual migraines. This class of medication is nonsedating, but GI upset is common. The usual dose is 500 to 550 mg once a day.

Combination drugs associated with migraine pain relief include Midrin, Fioricet, Esgic, and Firorinal. These contain varying combinations of a pain reliever (e.g., aspirin, acetaminophen), caffeine, sedating compounds, and vasoconstrictors. (Vasoconstrictors are sometimes used alone.)

Other drugs that are sometimes used in severe or prolonged headache cases include corticosteroids, DHE nasal spray, and Ketorolac (Toradol) injections.

OTC preparations that may relieve migraine pain include Excedrin Migraine and ibuprofen.

Migraine Prevention

Patients who suffer three or more migraine headaches a month may find that using medications to prevent the onset of the headache is the wisest strategy. Medications may be combined in some cases. Many drugs found to be useful for preventing migraine headaches were developed for other purposes.

Originally developed as an antiseizure medication, Depakote (valproate) is now frequently used to prevent migraine headaches, but may take four to six weeks to become effective. Side effects include lethargy, depression, GI upset, and difficulties with memory. Topamax (topiramate) and Neurontin (gabapentin) are two additional antiseizure medications sometimes used to treat migraines.

Anti-inflammatories are sometimes used to treat and prevent migraine headaches. In the last few years, the newer anti-inflammatories developed to relieve pain caused by osteoarthritis and other bone and joint pain may be suggested for preventive purposes. These include the COX-2 inhibitors, marketed under the names Vioxx and Celebrex. These drugs are also nonsedating.

Two classes of drugs were designed to treat hypertension (elevated blood pressure) and heart disease:

1. Beta-blockers, (e.g., Lopressor [metoprolol] and Blocadren [timolol]). They are sometimes used in combination with amitriptyline (Elavil), which is an antidepressant.
2. Calcium channel blockers, (e.g., Calan [verapamil]).

Because of the risk of drug interaction it is important that your physician be aware of any medication you are taking for any purpose.

PROVIDING INFORMATION, ASKING QUESTIONS

When your physician suggests a medication to you it is your job to:

- report prior experience with the drug, including side effects you experienced;
- be certain your doctor knows if you are pregnant or breastfeeding, or may become pregnant;
- report all other prescription medications you are taking in order to avoid drug interactions;
- report all OTC medications and nutritional supplements you take (including any herbal formulations).

Make sure your physician explains these issues to your satisfaction:

- the correct dosage;
- what to do if you skip a dose or mistakenly take too much medication in one dose;
- what the expected side effects are, especially those that require you to immediately stop taking the medication;
- what to do in case of severe adverse reaction;
- what the best time of day is to take the medication and whether it should be taken on an empty or a full stomach;
- how to store the medication;
- how soon symptom relief should begin;
- what would be an alternative plan if the medication is ineffective;
- what are the possible effects on children or the elderly.

Glossary

Acute. An illness that begins quickly and produces a cluster of symptoms associated with the condition. With most infections, treatment and/or time resolves the symptoms while the body fights off the harmful invading organism.

Adenoids. Lymph tissue in the nasopharynx designed to help fight infection, but which can cause respiratory difficulties in children. Adenoidal tissues usually shrink in adolescence. The adenoids are sometimes removed during a tonsillectomy (the surgical procedure that removes the tonsils).

Ageusia. Inability to taste.

Allergy. The overreaction of the immune system to an allergen, which is any substance that triggers an allergic reaction in the body.

Analgesic. A pain-relieving substance.

Anaphylaxis. The extreme allergic response that can quickly close airways and become life threatening. Requires immediate epinephrine injection to counteract the body's overreaction to an allergen.

Anosmia. The inability to smell, either temporarily or permanently.

Antibiotics. Several families of medication designed to fight bacterial infections—ineffective against viruses that may produce similar symptoms.

Antibodies. Proteins called immunoglobulins produced as a defensive mechanism to neutralize proteins that are foreign to the body.

Antitussive. Medication given to relieve coughing.

Apnea. A condition characterized by cessation of breathing, often occurring during sleep.

Asthma. A respiratory disease that narrows the bronchi and causes sudden shortness of breath, coughing, and wheezing.

Aura. Sensory changes involving vision, taste, or smell that precede the onset of a classic migraine.

Bacteria. A group of microorganisms that cause acute infections and whose effects can be neutralized by the correct antibiotic medication.

Basophils. Cells that circulate in the bloodstream that are involved in allergic reactions (e.g., releasing histamine).

Bronchi. Tubes that go from the trachea into the lungs, which when narrowed produces a state of bronchoconstriction or blockage; abnormal contractions of the lung's airways are called bronchospasms.

Bronchodilator. A medication that widens the airways and is used to restore normal breathing during asthma attacks.

Chronic. Any condition in which treatment is incomplete and symptoms persist, or a condition that recurs on a regular basis and for which treatment results are variable.

Cilia. The tiny (microscopic) hairs that line the airways and propel mucus through the respiratory system.

Cluster headaches. One-sided headaches, usually intense, that may produce nasal or allergy symptoms and are triggered in a variety of ways.

Cold. The common name for an upper respiratory infection (UTI), which is usually caused by a rhinovirus.

Congestion. An accumulation of fluid that blocks normal movement of air through the nasal structures and into the lungs.

CT scan. Computerized tomography, an X-ray-imaging test that provides detailed information about the condition of organs and tissues.

Decongestant. Medications designed to act against nasal congestion and open the nasal passages. May be used in oral preparations or as a nasal spray.

Dysgeusia. Distorted perception of taste.

Dysomia. Distorted perception of odors.

Endoscope. Diagnostic and surgical tool that allows a magnified view of the sinuses and surgical field during the procedure called "endoscopy." ESS refers to endoscopic sinus surgery.

Eosinophils. A type of white blood cell involved in allergic responses and sinus diseases and may be involved in the body's response to fungal growth.

Expectorant. A type of cough medication designed to loosen and clear secretions from the bronchial tubes rather than suppressing the coughing reflex.

Gastroesophageal reflux disease. The "backup" or regurgitation of stomach acid and partially digested food into the esophagus. The irritation this causes my cause throat and bronchial irritation and mimic symptoms of sinusitis.

Gustation. The scientific term for the sense of taste.

Histamine. A substance produced in the body in response to exposure to an allergen that then triggers nasal and respiratory symptoms, itching, and watery eyes. Components of drugs (prescription and OTC) designed to counteract these symptoms are in a class of substances called antihistamines.

Hypergeusia. Increased ability to taste.

Hyperosmia. Abnormally sensitive sense of smell, usually associated with illnesses such as Addison's disease.

Hypogeusia. Subnormal sense of taste.

Hyposmia. Subnormal sense of smell caused by many conditions and diseases.

Immune system. Specialized cells and proteins whose primary job is protecting the body against potentially harmful foreign invaders such as bacteria, viruses, and fungi. It is sometimes described as an army that mobilizes to defend the body and maintain health. The symptoms produced when a person is exposed to an allergen are triggered by the immune system that misinterprets the substance as harmful. Immunotherapy is a type of allergy treatment that attempts to desensitize the individual to the allergen, thereby preventing the symptoms. Immunoassays are the tests used to investigate the invading organisms and the body's response to them. The terms *immunodeficient* or *immunosuppressed* apply to conditions in which the immune system fails to protect the body against disease. HIV/AIDS and chemotherapy treatment can lead to immunosuppression.

Immunoglobulins. Proteins in the blood we also call *antibodies*; during an allergic reaction the body produces immunoglobulin E (IgE).

Inflammation. The general term used for a localized reaction to irritation or injury or by "foreign invaders" such as virus and bacteria. The affected tissues may appear red and/or swollen.

Mast cells. Cells that contain histamine that are found in mucous membranes in the respiratory tract. These cells are involved in allergic responses.

Migraine. One-sided and severe headache associated with an imbalance of neurotransmitters in the brain and triggered in a variety of ways. *Migraineurs* is a term used to identify patients who suffer frequent migraine headaches or are susceptible to them. Classic migraines are preceded by sensory changes, (e.g., phantom odors); common migraines often involve nausea and vomiting.

MRI (magnetic resonance imaging). A diagnostic test that does not use radiation and is now used to image various structures in the body.

Mucokinetic/mucolytic. Pertains to agents that thin mucus, thus allowing it to flow through the respiratory tract.

Mucous membrane. The soft tissues that line many structures in the body; these membranes secrete mucus, which is one of the immune system's weapons to prevent invading substances from harming the body.

Nasal cycle. The change in size and shape of the inside of the nose that occurs naturally several times a day.

NSAIDs (non-steroidal anti-inflammatory drugs). Drugs that act as analgesics and are frequently used to relieve headache pain and symptoms associated with sinus infections and colds. They are also a class of analgesics that do not contain aspirin.

Obstructive sleep apnea (OSA). During sleep, a temporary blockage of the oropharynx that obstructs the normal flow of air into the lungs. This causes a decrease in the blood and brain, snoring, frequent awakenings through the night, and a feeling of fatigue during the day.

Olfaction. The scientific word for the sense of smell.

Olfactory cycle. The naturally occurring change in the concentration of odor molecules that reach the top of the nose through one or the other nostril. This is experienced as a subtle difference in congestion in each nostril, and olfactory ability is greater in the more congested nostril.

Olfactory epithelia. Mucus-coated membranes and the site at which air currents develop and allow higher concentrations of odor molecules to be processed and experienced as smells.

Olfactory membrane. An area about the size of the head of a pin that functions as a central processing plant for odor molecules.

Olfactory receptors. Millions of sites located on the olfactory nerve; these receptors help identify and distinguish odors.

Ostia. The opening of the sinus through which mucus drains into the nose. The ostiomeatal complex is the area into which all the sinuses drain; blockage reduces or prevents draining of other sinus cavities, thus creating conditions in which infections can develop.

OTC (over the counter). Medications available without prescription.

Pansinusitis. A sinus infection involving all the sinus cavities.

Paranasal sinuses. The sinuses close to the nasal cavity.

Pathogen. Any bacteria, virus, fungus, or other foreign microorganism that can cause disease in the body.

Perennial allergies. Allergies to environmental or food substances that are present throughout the year.

Phantageusia. Perception of a taste that isn't there or a hallucinated taste.

Phantosmia. Perception of an odor that isn't there, or a hallucinated smell.

Placebo effect. The effect of an inactive substance, usually called a "sugar pill," used in scientific studies to investigate the efficacy of an active substance, usually a drug. The belief or assumption that the substance has an effect on the body produces the effect.

Polyps. Small benign tissues that arise from mucous membranes which may block nasal passages and impair olfactory ability. They are called "growths," but they actually have the same cell structure as the tissue from which they appear.

Purulent. A "fancy" name for pus, which is the liquid product of infection; it contains white blood cells, dead tissue, microorganisms, and so forth, and ranges in color from clear to white to yellow to green.

Rhinitis. Medical term for nasal congestion or runny nose. *Rhino* refers to the nose; *itis* is the medical suffix that means inflammation.

Seasonal allergies. Allergies to substances that occur in seasonal cycles.

Sinus headaches. A misnomer for perceived pressure and pain in the sinuses, but which may be another type of headache, or caused by pain originating in the turbinates or ostia.

Steroids (also called corticosteroids or cortisone). The shortened term for the synthetically produced version of hormones secreted by the adrenal glands. Steroid medications for sinus conditions are used both orally and in nasal sprays; this class of medication is also prepared for use by injection and in ointments.

Tension headaches. Believed to be caused by stress, specifically the muscle contractions resulting from stress, but that may ultimately be traced to dental malocclusion that subtly distorts the pathway of the temporomandibular joint (TMJ) and causes the pain that may affect the whole head, the neck, and the shoulders.

Tic douloureux. Sudden severe pain in the face that is spasmodic in nature; the condition is also known as *trigeminal neuralgia*.

Tonsils. Tissue at the back of the throat involved in fighting infection in one's early years. They can become infected and cause numerous symptoms; at one time they were routinely removed in childhood.

Turbinates. Structures in the nose that are covered by a mucous membrane that may swell and obstruct breathing and the flow of mucus.

Bibliography

Balk, Ethan M., et al. "Strategies for Diagnosing and Treating Suspected Acute Bacterial Sinusitis: A Cost-effective Analysis." *Journal of General Internal Medicine* (Oct. 2001); 16 (10): 701–711.

Black, W. D. "The Diagnosis of Headache of Nasal Origin." *Southern Medical Journal* (March 1921); XIV: 3: 242–246.

Blumenthal, Harvey J. "Headaches and Sinus Disease." *Headache* (Oct. 2001); 41: 9: 883–838.

Cady, Roger K., and Curtis P. Schreiber. "Sinus Headache or Migraine? Considerations in Making a Differential Diagnosis." *Neurology* (May 2002); 58 (9 Suppl 6): S10–S14.

Casale, Thomas B., et al. "Effect of Omalizumab on Symptoms of Seasonal Allergic Rhinitis. *Journal of the American Medical Association (JAMA)* (Dec. 19, 2001); 286: 23: 2956–2967.

Couch, James R. "Sinus Headache: A Neurologist's Viewpoint." *Seminars in Neurology* (Dec. 1988); 8: 4: 298–302.

Davidson, Terence M., et al. "Smell Impairment: Can It Be Reversed?" *Postgraduate Medicine* (July 1995); 98: 1: 107–109, 112–118.

Davies, Andrew, et al. "The Effect of Acupuncture on Nonallergic Rhinitis: A Controlled Pilot Study." *Alternative Therapies in Health and Medicine* (Jan. 1998); 4: 70–74.

DeCook, C. A., and A. R. Hirsch. "Anosmia Due to Inhalational Zinc: A Case Report." *Chemical Senses* (2000); 25: 5: 659.

Diagnosis and Treatment of Acute Bacterial Rhinosinusitis. AHCPR: Evidence Report/Technology Assessment Number Nine (March 1999); Publication No. 99–E016.

Dolor, Rowena, et al. "Comparison of Cefuroxime with or Without Intranasal Fluticasone for the Treatment of Rhinosinusitis." *JAMA* (Dec. 26, 2001); 286: 24: 3097–3105.

Goldman, George E., et al. "Isolated Sphenoid Sinusitis." *American Journal of Emergency Medicine* (May 1993); 3: 235–238.

Hirsch, Alan R. "Aromatherapy: Art, Science, or Myth?" Weintraub MI (Ed.), In: *Alternative and Complementary Treatment in Neurologic Illness*, Philadelphia, PA: Churchill Livingstone, 2001, pp.128–150.

———"Negative Health Effects of Malodors in the Environment." *Journal of Neurol Orthop Med Surg* (1998); 18: 43–45.

———"Olfactory Dysfunction as a Symptom in Various Conditions." *Journal Neurol Orthop Med Surg* (Nov. 4, 1992); 13: 4: 298–302.

———"Olfaction in Migraineurs." *Headache* (May 1992); 32: 5: 233–236.

Hirsch, Alan R., and Maria L. Colavincenzo. "Olfactory Deficits Among Chicago Firefighters." *Chicago Medicine* (Nov. 2000); 103: 11: 18–19.

———"Failure of Physicians to Assess Olfactory Ability in Neurologic Inpatients." *Chemical Senses* (1999); 24: 5: 607–608.

Ikeda, Katsuhisa, et al. "Efficacy of Systemic Corticosteroid Treatment for Anosmia with Nasal and Paranasal Sinus Disease." *Rhinology* (1994); 33: 162–165.

Jafek, B. W. "Biopsies of Human Olfactory Epithelium." *Chemical Senses* (2002); 27: 7: 623–628.

Jonas, Wayne B. "A Critical Overview of Homeopathy." *Annals of Internal Medicine* (March 4, 2003); 138: 5: 393–399.

Leopold, Donald A. "Nasal Toxicity: End Points of Concern in Humans." *Inhalation Toxicology* (1994); 6: 23–29.

"Local Transmission of Plasmodium *vivax malaria*—Virginia 2002." From the Centers for Disease Control and Prevention. *JAMA* (Nov. 6, 2002); 288: 17: 2113–2114.

Lund, V. J. "Heath Related Quality of Life in Sinonasal Disease." *Rhinology* (2001); 39: 4: 182–186.

Semchenko, A., et al. "Management of Acute Sinusitis and Acute Otitis Media." AFP Monograph (Jan. 2001); 1.

Naclerio, Robert. "Diagnosis and Management of Chronic Sinusitis." *Clinical Comment* (Jan. 1995); 12: 1: 1–3.

Plaut, Marshall. "Immune-Based Targeted Therapy for Allergic Diseases." *JAMA* (Dec. 19, 2001); 286: 3005–3006.

"Practical Solutions for Medical Treatment Failures: A Case-Based Analysis." (Based on a presentation by Paul Winner), *Proceedings: Advanced Studies in Medicine* (March 2003); 3: 38: S164–S167.

Ratner, Paul H., et al. "Use of Intranasal Cromolyn Sodium for Allergic Rhinitis." *Mayo Clinic Proceedings* (April 2002); 77: 4: 350–354.

Saper, Joel. "Chronic Daily Headache: A Clinician's Perspective." *Headache: The Journal of Head and Face Pain* (June 2002); 42: 6: 538.

Seiden, Allen M. "Olfactory Loss Secondary to Nasal and Sinus Pathology." In: Seiden AM (Ed). *Taste and Smell Disorders* (New York: Thieme, 1997); 52–71.

Skoner, David P. "Complications of Allergic Rhinitis." *Journal of Allergy and Clinical Immunology* (June 2000); 105: 6 (Pt. 2): S605–S609.

Sonnenschein, Robert. "Headaches: With Special Reference to Those of Nasal Origin." *Illinois Medical Journal* (Oct. 1920); 38: 315–318.

van Buchem, F. L.; et al. "Primary-Care-Based Randomised Placebo-Controlled Trial of Antibiotic Treatment in Acute Maxillary Sinusitis." *The Lancet* (March 8, 1997); 349: 683–687.

Willett, Laura Rees, et al. "Current Diagnosis and Management of Sinusitis." *Journal of General Internal Medicine* (Jan. 1994); 9: 1: 38–45.

Wilson, William R., and William W. Montgomery. "Infectious Diseases of the Paranasal Sinuses." Paparella M. M., Shumrick D. A., Gluckman J. L., Meyerhoff W. L. (Eds.). In: *Otolaryngology, Volume III: Head and Neck, Third Edition.* Philadelphia, PA: Saunders (1991); 1843–1860.

Wolfensberger, Markus, and Thomas Hummel. "Anti-Inflammatory and Surgical Therapy of Olfactory Disorders Related to Sino-Nasal Disease." *Chemical Senses* (2002); 27: 7: 617–622.

Index

Symptoms (*cont.*)
in children, 184–85
chronic sinusitis, 55–57
colds, 18–26, 23
fighting your, 26–28
GERD, 58–59
migraine headaches, 100–102, 197
sinusitis versus colds, 19, 21–22, 39–41

Taste, 104–5, 111–13
Taste disorders, xvii–xix, 104–6, 113
Tavist, 205
T cells, 65, 151, 182
Tear gas, 112
Temporomandibular joint dysfunction (TMJ), 91–92
Tension headaches, 84–86, 89, 218
Tests
for allergies, 71–72, 181
for headaches, 102–3
for immune system, 194–95
for smell loss, 128–29
Thyroid replacement treatment, 114
Tic douloureux, 92–93, 218
Tiger Balm, 142
Time management, 166
Tonsillectomy, 188
Tonsils, 182, 188, 218
Toxic fumes, 121–23, 135, 136, 158
Treatment. *See also* Self-care strategies; *and specific treatments*
acute sinusitis, 43–45
allergies, 71–76, 77–78, 204–6
of children, 185–87
chronic sinusitis, 52–53, 56–57, 77–78
colds, 26–36, 200–206
cost-effective, xix–xxii
medications guide, 199–211
migraine headaches, 99–100, 190–91, 208–10

smell loss, 126–28
Triaminic, 200
Trichloroethylene, 123
Trigeminal nerve, 92–93, 95–96, 112
Triptans, 208–9
Turbinate hypertrophy, 173
Turbinates, 6–9, 13–14
defined, 218
pain and, 15–17
surgery and, 171, 173–74, 176–77
Turbinitis, 16–17
Tylenol, 33, 186, 202
Tyramine, 98

Upper respiratory tract infections (URI), 64
Urinary tract infections, 80

Valproate, 209–10
Vaporizers, 27, 141, 186
Vasoconstrictors, 209
Vicks, 142, 201, 203
Vicodin, 209
Viral rhinitis. *See* Colds
Vitamin A, 150
Vitamin C, 150–51
colds and, 29, 30–31
Vitamin E, 150, 151

Water, 139–42
Water park sinus congestion, 133–34
White blood cells, 24, 30
Winter cold season, 23–25

Yogurt, 206

Zicam, 34–35
Zinc (zinc lozenges), 33–34, 35, 150, 151
Zyrtec, 73, 205

About the Author

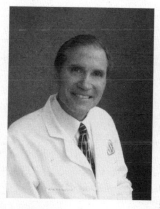

Well-known neurologist and psychiatrist Alan Hirsch, M.D., F.A.C.P., developed an interest in smell and taste when, during his medical school years, he sustained a minor head injury and for a period of time smelled everything in his environment like cigarette smoke, even when no one was smoking. He quickly learned that our ability to smell is the most forgotten sense, and in 1984 he founded the Smell & Taste Treatment and Research Foundation in Chicago, Illinois. Through his work he has educated the public about the importance of the sense of smell and its partner, the sense of taste, and the health consequences when these senses are impaired.

Dr. Hirsch has conducted dozens of studies about the role of smell and taste in human health and society. His work has explained the relationship between smell and weight loss, sexual arousal and attraction, personality traits, human communication, and even the way this sense influences marketing and sales. While his scientific work is serious and has important implications for health and culture, Dr. Hirsch also brings a sense of humor to his frequent media appearances. He has been a guest on *The Oprah Winfrey Show,* CNN, National Public Radio, *Good Morning America, Dateline,* and many other national programs, and his work has been featured in diverse newspapers and magazines including *The New York Times, Redbook,* and *Cosmopolitan.*

Dr. Hirsch is an assistant professor in the departments of neurology and psychiatry at Rush University Medical Center in Chicago.

OTHER TITLES FROM THE BESTSELLING SERIES
WHAT YOUR DOCTOR MAY *NOT* TELL YOU ABOUT™...

AUTOIMMUNE DISORDERS
The Revolutionary Drug-free Treatments for Thyroid
Disease • Lupus • MS • IBD • Chronic Fatigue •
Rheumatoid Arthritis, and Other Diseases

BREAST CANCER
How Hormone Balance Can Help Save Your Life

CHILDREN'S ALLERGIES AND ASTHMA
Simple Steps to Help Stop Attacks and Improve Your
Child's Health

CHILDREN'S VACCINATIONS
Learn What You Should—and Should Not—Do to Protect
Your Kids

CIRCUMCISION
Untold Facts on America's Most Widely Performed—and
Most Unnecessary—Surgery

FIBROIDS
New Techniques and Therapies—Including
Breakthrough Alternatives

FIBROMYALGIA
The Revolutionary Treatment That Can Reverse
the Disease

FIBROMYALGIA FATIGUE
The Powerful Program That Helps You Boost Your Energy
and Reclaim Your Life

more...

HIP AND KNEE REPLACEMENT SURGERY
Everything You Need to Know to Make the Right Decisions

HPV AND ABNORMAL PAP SMEARS
Get the Facts on This Dangerous Virus—Protect Your Health and Your Life!

HYPERTENSION
The Revolutionary Nutrition and Lifestyle Program to Help Fight High Blood Pressure

HYPOTHYROIDISM
A Simple Plan for Extraordinary Results

KNEE PAIN AND SURGERY
Learn the Truth About MRIs and Common Misdiagnoses— and Avoid Unnecessary Surgery

MENOPAUSE
The Breakthrough Book on *Natural* Hormone Balance

MIGRAINES
The Breakthrough Program That Can Help End Your Pain

OSTEOPOROSIS
Help Prevent—and Even Reverse—the Disease That Burdens Millions of Women

PARKINSON'S DISEASE
A Holistic Program for Optimal Wellness

PEDIATRIC FIBROMYALGIA
A Safe, New Treatment Plan for Children

PREMENOPAUSE
Balance Your Hormones and Your Life from Thirty to Fifty